LAB VALUES

An Easy Guide to Learn Everything You Need to Know About Laboratory Medicine and its Importance in Diagnosing Disease

By

Nathan Orwell

Legal Notice:

Discover the Entire Collection!

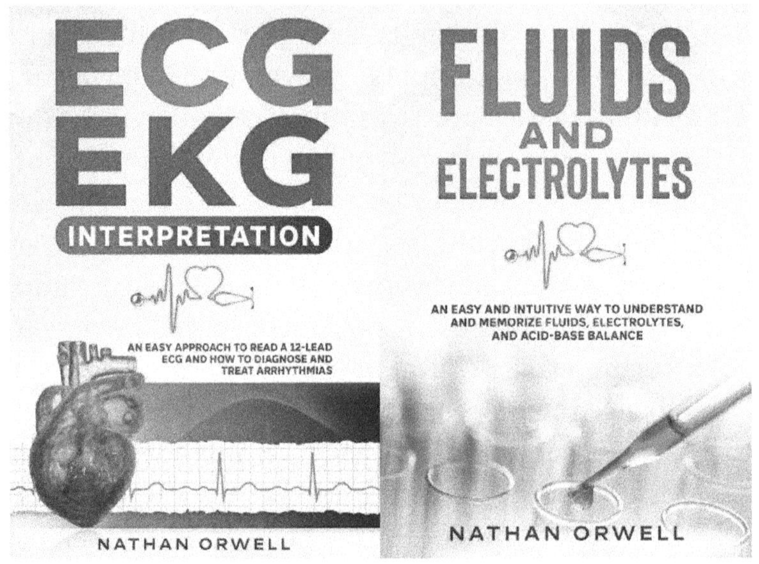

Table of Contents

Introduction

The primary things that affect all medical approaches in various diversification are the right knowledge of laboratory tests or values. When a patient is sick, the first thing needed to be done is to run a test to confirm the assumption from all the symptoms noticed so far. Although the need for laboratory tests and values cannot be limited in the medical field, the practitioners are not given the right regards on their works. And this is affecting the medical world, as far as medicine is concerned.

This book is enlightening and will help you see the medical world from another angle. First, as a medical student, it will show you the need to put your eye on laboratory details and values. The book would give you the importance and reasons to stand out among your colleagues — just by observing the little things they might not put in mind.

As far as medical laboratory tests and values are concerned. It cannot be argued that the uniqueness of laboratory tests is the same reason it is required at an early stage of all medical practice. The test can give useful insights on the things to look for; what is affecting the patient, what to use, and many more in medical practices.

Looking at results is the other complementary thing to the initial practices about laboratory tests. And this includes sample collection, sample preparation, sample handling, among others.

The most advantageous way of using this book is by observing the crucial ends of each chapter and noting the significant differences in each chapter that are unique to the laboratory and medical world at large. All in all, values are important. And all the results from each section are based on values!

Chapter 1: Overview of Laboratory Samples

The only thing that is important in all the processes involved in performing laboratory tests is the **values**. When a medical officer has the right values, he/she is able to perform all medical procedures, diagnosis, and administration of drugs or prescriptions.

What is a value then?

Value is the main thing that gives meaning to all the things medical personnel will do after accessing the patient. Firstly, the medical provider knows that the patient is either sick or has an issue. And the next step is to assess the situation via the laboratory technician as they would give reports on the findings, which indicates *"what is wrong."* The feedback on what is precisely wrong with the person is the value that saves a life. So, without the values, medical personnel may not perform his/her respective field in an excellent manner.

The significance of value is the biochemical importance in it. We live on both system and molecular levels. A sick body is not fit from the molecular level, and it is noticed at the systemic level.

So, the values give the biochemical processes that fire on in the patient, and medical personnel can build on it.

From the little expression above, the process is not simple at all. Although it might not go past the act of a nurse extracting blood samples from a patient, it is more difficult in the **sense of errors**. If errors are equipped in the values, it is enough to cause complications and may even lead to death. Sometimes, the overall tests may indicate "YES/NO" values — An example is a test for HIV. Wrong approaches would definitely cause complications, and there is a need to prevent that no matter what.

Start by giving regards to each process involved in drawing samples, observing, and running several tests. Another important thing is to make each stage meaningful - all in all, life is involved. Then, take a right eye on each step involved in collecting laboratory data, diagnosis, and treatment.

1.1 Samples Come Naturally from the body

Overview

Samples are all over our bodies. As medical practitioners or students. It is necessary to know all the places and types of the sample that can be extracted from each location. And another thing is the difference in removing the same samples from more than one location. For example, samples from the urine and blood can be used to carry out glucose testing. Notwithstanding, they have different significances – *while blood glucose tests are more suitable to blood samples, urinalysis is significant to the urine sample*. The main thing is to know the reason for extracting samples from a considerable location.

Today, the collection of samples is more straightforward and may vary from **patient approaches** (which requires little to zero medical assistance) to **medical professionals**. Before now, a patient may be given a sample bottle to take a sample at home and bring it to the hospital on the next appointment. However, it is not common nowadays. The majority of toilets in the hospitals have slots to take samples and well comprehensive instructions on the walls.

This minimizes the patient interaction with the samples and therefore improves the accuracy of the values.

Now, either patients take samples on their own or via the assistant of medical personnel; people involved should try as much as possible to prevent any act that contaminates the sample. First of all, let us discuss ***the type of samples and how to avoid contamination.***

Examples of types of samples collected by the patient

Firstly, all patients must understand the process involved in taking their samples, followed by a thorough examination of the act to prevent contamination.

Examples

1) **Semen**

The male patient ejaculates into a sample container. It is highly prioritized that the patient refrains from sex or forms of ejaculation for at least 2 days before the test. During the process, condoms, lubricants, or forms of contaminates should be avoided.

The aim is to get pure samples that carry a significant percentage of the right values. The sample should be delivered within 1 hour of extraction. In all conditions, it must be kept very close to body temperature and must not be either frozen or refrigerated.

2) Sputum

Sputum is first taken early in the morning before anything. Most of the time, patients can easily take the sample by themselves by coughing from deep down their lungs. It is considered to be more advantageous if the patient does not eat any food. It is expected that the sputum is relatively thin, unlike the usually watery one that has been mixed with saliva.

3) Stool

Patients often take these samples themselves just by observing the necessary things in the toilet. On the choice of test, patients may be instructed to collect the piece by smearing a small amount on or scooping a small portion into a vial, a container, or a particular test paper. All in all, it is expected to follow the regular instructions to prevent contamination in any means.

4) Urine

Urine is directly taken by the patient unless in a urinary catheter, which requires medical assistance. Often, the patient is expected to observe specific measures to prevent contamination outside the body — the patient may need to clean the outer body and release a bit of the urine before taking it into the container.

5) Saliva

Saliva collection varies depending on the quantity required. A swab is enough for a small amount of saliva, and a large portion might demand continuous release into the container without producing sputum.

Examples of types of samples collected from within

Some samples cannot be reached without piercing the body. The process to collect these samples may be painful or, at least, makes the patient a little bit uncomfortable. Aside from this, they are carried out by practitioners — a nurse, phlebotomist, or trained medical officer. All in all, the extractor needs to follow specific procedures to keep the samples safe for exact values.

Another case is the need for an anesthetic to keep the patient in control. This process is complicated, especially the ones that are related to cerebral fluids.

Examples

1) **Blood**

Blood samples vary in extraction. Some are just a drop, and some are taken by suctioning. The common thing is that it is carried out by phlebotomists or medical personnel. The procedure is a short time process and it is slightly painful, especially at inserting the needle and post-extraction.

2) **Tissue Biopsy**

Tests of tissue might be acquired from various diverse body locales, for example, lung, lymph, or skin. Contingent upon the site and the level of intrusiveness, some pain or inconvenience may happen. The time needed to play out the methodology and for recuperation can likewise shift significantly. These processes are led by medical care practitioners who have had specific training. The process is in two types:

***Needle biopsy**: needle is inserted into the place, and extract fluid from the location. It is slightly painful, and a simple pinch may be experienced. The patient may observe pains after the extraction.*

Excisional biopsy*: this is minor surgery to obtain the right sample from the inner tissue. This time, an incision is made, and a bit of the tissue is extracted from the body.*

3) Cerebrospinal fluid

This is one of the most advanced sample taking. It is performed by using special needles like a spinal tap. Often, the needle is inserted into the spinal between two vertebrae. Pain and discomfort are expected to rush in after the process.

1.2 Sampling and Preparation for Laboratory Values

Overview

There are various means of gathering information on a patient, and one of the ways is sampling, which is used in order to generate laboratory values. In all these preparation processes, there are five vital/main stages a sample must pass through before it is finalized to exist as a sample. Any handler or medical personnel must know the importance of each step and get the right knowledge to make the sample survive the stages without causing any damage to the samples.

As discussed earlier, a sample can be a simple body fluid gotten from a single swab; it can also be a tissue extracted from minor surgical procedures. All in all, medical practitioners must be familiar with the five stages.

The five crucial stages involved in sampling are the following: **sample preparation, sample collection, sample handling, sample transportation, and sample storage.**

1. Sample Preparation

Sample preparation is the elementary stage that precedes all other steps. This is the stage where the patient is screened to know if he/she is fit for the task ahead. Several things are put into practice to tell if a patient should move further or not. *For example, the sample preparation for an aged-adult above 70 is different from a kid below 12 years.* The medical personnel may check weight, age, and type of condition to know the right step in the hierarchy. The crucial end of sample preparation is documentation. It is possible that the same practitioners that obtained the values for the sample preparation may not carry out the sample collection, sample transportation, and some other stages. So, documentation is highly crucial.

Additionally, the patient must be confirmed as the right person for the process before sample collection can take place. For example, through a thorough identifying mode that will check the patient's name (maybe by asking or asking his/her family) and checked against the patient tag as the case may be.

This is the stage to confirm if the patient needs to perform some actions such as *"using a drug before the sample is taken, or if fasting is part of the prior preparation to make the sample ready for extraction."*

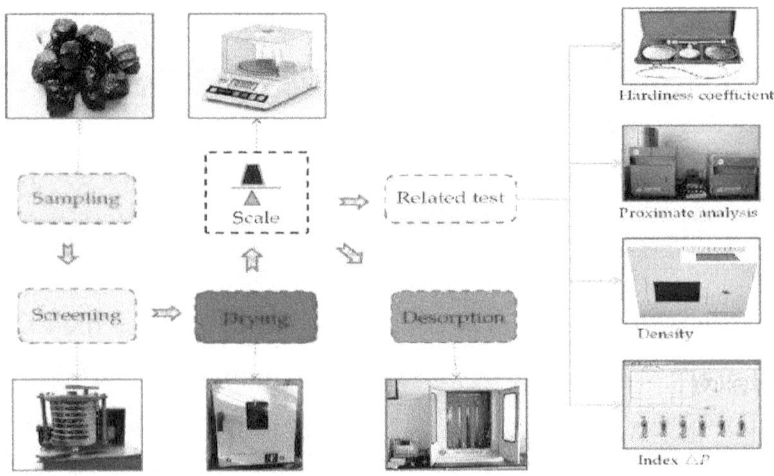

2. Sample collection

Sample collection is the main thing that surrounds all about sampling. At this point, the values obtained from "sample preparation" are used to collect the sample. From the prepared data, it will be known if the sample should be in large or small quantities. Additionally, the right location to obtain the samples would be known as well. Remember that there are various places to get samples, and each has significant importance.

If samples are wrongly collected, the laboratory values are meaningless. Look out for details and put yourself through thorough labeling. The process of labeling might be disturbing and uneasy if there are lots of samples to collect. Notwithstanding, the job has to be done.

Also, the sampling protocol must be clarified. Either the patient is obtaining the sample by him/herself or via the assistant of medical personnel; it all required the activation of the sampling protocol as this is the right way to prevent mistakes in any areas. Also, the sample must be arranged or collected to be easily identified–things like the name of the sample, date of receipt in the laboratory sample code number, and the like must be included as a permanent label to the sample.

3. Sample Handling

The first protocol of sample handling is to protect the sample from changes in composition and contamination. All the processes mentioned so far can be smooth, and the sample may be contaminated easily via wrong sample handling. In other words, it is straightforward to contaminate samples via the process of sample handling.

Before further processing, you must have all the knowledge to handle a sample. Mostly, sample handling is carried out by laboratory technicians. It is expected to have the best experience in the field, as various pieces demand unique steps to excellent handling. While some are needed to keep at a particular temperature, others may be handled like typical samples.

The handler needs to be aware of certain things while handling the sample.

- *Measurements or values before and after the process*
- *The suitable method to carry out the process to obtain exact values*
- *Weight, composition, and nature of the sample before further processing*
- *Apparatuses needed to carry out the test on the sample.*

4. Sample Transportation

Another crucial stage is transporting the sample. Even if the medical individual collected the piece with good reviews and obeyed all the protocols, it might be contaminated via wrong transportation. *For example, the smallest collection from the inner body of the patient should be kept at body temperature.* And any form of transportation should give the sample temperature environment to the sample.

Some transportation mediums can be sterilized materials, mini freezers, boxes, bags, cans. First, any medical personnel should keep a close eye on the sample and make sure it is in the best state in temperature, values. Also, the patient must be warned to observe all the processes as crucial ends to excellent results or contaminated ones. Blood, urine, and semen can be transported in a can or container; they should be kept at body temperature. Tissues gotten from a biopsy can be transported via boxes or mini freezer; the temperature should also be regulated to be in its best state.

Some of the things to consider while transporting a sample:

- *If the sample is bulky, the choice of transportation must be considered suitable before using any means to transport the material.*

- *Try to deliver samples to the laboratory promptly with the original conditions maintained as much as possible. And this falls in the hand of the medical handler and patient.*

- *The container or transporting medium must be clean, dry, leak-proof, airtight, sterile, suitable for the samples, as the case may be.*

5. Sample Storing

Each sample has unique places in which they are stored. Most practitioners do make the mistake of discarding pieces after obtaining the values. However, the professional approach demands a little storage even after performing and getting values from the samples. Another case is to store the processed sample when the test has been carried out; some samples are to be kept for reference purposes.

Keep samples in sample boxes that are air tight and leak-proof. If samples are not analyzed immediately, they should be left in cold storage to minimize spoilage and some other chemical reactions. Light may affect some samples; it is necessary to be stored in the dark.

Effects of sample storage, potential changes, and precautions:

Effects	**Potential Changes**	**Precaution**
Drying out	Due to loss of water	Use designed and verified protocol. Follow the instructions needed in order to perform clean sample extraction and handling. Weigh sample before and after each process (if needed).

Absorption	Sample gains more water	Use designed and verified protocol. Keep samples in an airtight or sealed container
Microbial activity	Degradation/autolysis/synthesis	Storage at low temperature. Keep at body temperature. Perform the procedure less than 60 minutes after extraction
Oxidation	Destruction of unsaturated fatty acids, loss of vitamins	Store at -3°C in a sealed container. Perform the procedure less than 60 minutes after extraction
Acid	Hydrolysis	Store at low temperatures

1.3 Blood Specimen Collection and Processing

Obtaining blood samples from a patient is a critical stage in the medical field, and it might lead to complicated conditions in case it is not done correctly. And this is why **phlebotomy** remains essential for various medical approaches, diagnoses, procedures, and tests. Although phlebotomy is not being taught in nursing school, all medical students must know the process. And this requires nursing students to go the extra mile in studying the procedure.

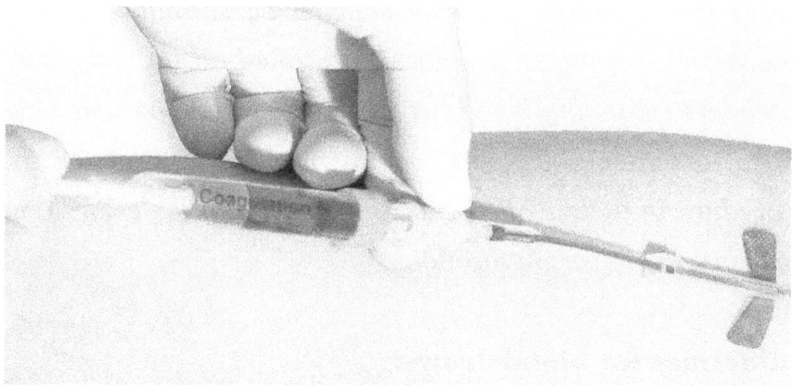

Most hospitals have phlebotomy teams; it is not an excuse to develop this skill because the staff in most hospitals is required to know everything about phlebotomy as the case may be.

Often, phlebotomy teams go on rounds in the hospital, and if an urgent test is called for, it is the duty of the nurse or medical personnel on duty to take the needed sample and perform the procedure.

As much as the course is not taught in nursing school, it is mandatory they study books and observed licensed nurses in clinical settings—on how they carried out the procedures. Notwithstanding, this book will put them through the process and make it easier to digest phlebotomy, but physical learning is mandatory.

Note: *phlebotomy cannot be learned by simply watching videos and step-by-step guides to fulfilled all the processes involved in drawing blood. In other words, you cannot read books to digest phlebotomy or to practice it. Practice the procedure in a controlled environment full of superiors and supervisors to put you through.*

Guidelines for blood draws:

- *Planning ahead*
- *Using an appropriate location*
- *Quality control*

Patient care for hospitals to adhere by:

- *Appropriate training in phlebotomy*
- *Cooperation on the part of patients*
- *Quality of laboratory sampling*
- *Availability of post-exposure prophylaxis (PEP)*
- *Availability of appropriate supplies and protective equipment*
- *Avoidance of contaminated phlebotomy equipment*

Steps in Drawing Blood Correctly

Step 1: Identify the vein

The first thing to know is the vein to puncture, and this varies from adult to young patient. In an adult patient, the common veins are the **median cubital vein** located in the antecubital fossa. This vein can also be called VC, and it is commonly referred to as antecubital. It can be found in the elbow's crevice between the median cephalic and the median basilica vein.

The median cubital vein is large, and it can yield excess blood if it is punctured wrongly or with a wide opening. Likewise, **peripheral intravenous catheters** are used to regulate the blood flow and can also be used to obtain frequent blood. So, if large quantities of blood samples are needed, a catheter may be suitable in that sense.

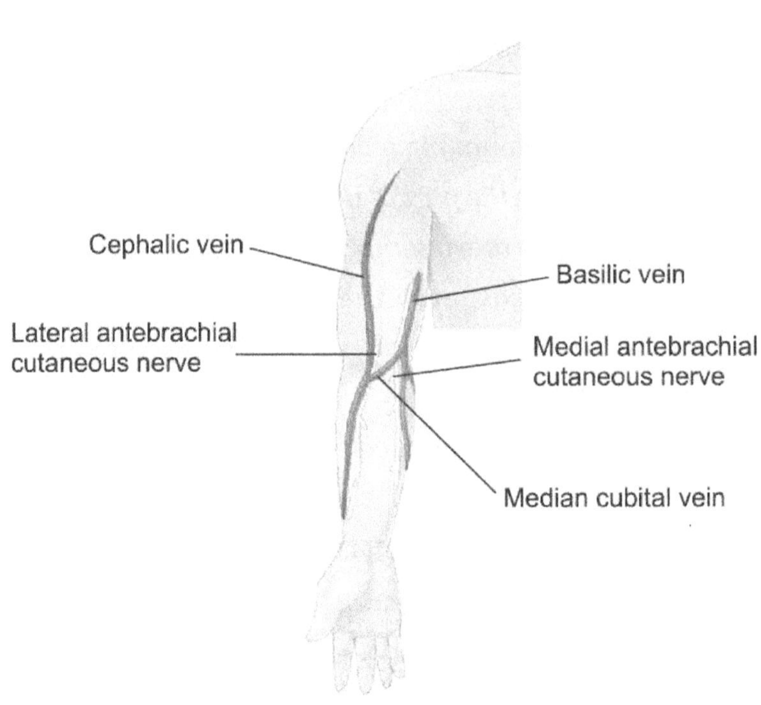

Although other commonly used veins are **basilic vein and cephalic vein,** the median cubital vein is widely used for beginner's phlebotomists because it is close to the skin and does not turn when punctured. In addition, it has a low risk of causing complications while extracting blood. Notwithstanding, it is expected to know all the anatomy of the prominent veins and arteries to master all the body systems and become an expert in phlebotomy. In other words, understanding the interaction between basilic vein, cephalic vein, and median cubital vein does not make an expert phlebotomist.

As much as you know where to puncture, you should see the place to avoid while performing the process. And the places to avoid are more than the location of the puncture. Knowing the "do and don't" definitely pushes you forward to become an expert in the field.

Some of the areas are listed below.

- The arm on a mastectomy
- Edematous locales
- Scarred part
- Arm with a prior or current blood cluster
- Fistulas
- Destinations over an IV cannula in a similar vessel
- Arm with PICC line
- Hematomas
- From an IV cannula (except if allowed by your foundation
- By means of an open injury or zone of contamination
- Arm in which blood is being bonded
- The arm on a surgery

Step 2: Gather Supplies

Once the location and vein are identified, the next step is to gather the necessary supplies. Some institution or hospital may have all the stores in a kit, and some others might require the handler to pick them individually. Whichever way, try to take extra kits with you. Some cases may require **second venipuncture**, and the needed materials must be ready to prevent complications.

Some of the necessary tools include:

- Appropriate blood-drawing needles
- Bio-hazard leak-proof transportation bags
- Puncture resistant sharps container
- Tourniquet
- Blood transfer device
- Adhesive bandage/tape
- Hand Sanitizer
- Alcohol swabs for skin disinfection
- Evacuated Collection Tubes (tubes which are specific to labs ordered)
- Personal Protective Equipment (i.e., gloves)
- Laboratory specimen labels
- Gauze
- Laboratory forms

Blood Specimen Collection Procedures

Venipuncture procedure

1. The first thing is to identify the patient and confirm it positively. Ask the patient his/her name by pronouncing and spelling it. Then, check it against the database or tag as the case may be.
2. Explain the procedure and reason for the blood-draw to the patient. Check the requisition form or any paperwork to confirm patient information or any special draw requirements. Sample extraction is now in a different stage; try to establish all the previous steps like *sample preparation* before collecting the sample such as checking for any *sensitivities or allergies with the patient as regards adhesives, latex, or antiseptics. An allergy ID band should be used to identify true allergies, but sensitivities may not be reported at the time of patient admission.*

3. Gather the necessary supplies that would be needed through the process

4. Place the patient in a sitting or lying position

5. Wash your hands, and disinfect if needed.

6. Mark the best position for venipuncture, and place the tourniquet 3 or 4 inches above the marked area.

7. Avoid the tourniquet to exceed 1 minute after inserting. Also, do not put it on too tight.

8. Use non-latex gloves and palpate for a vein.

9. After selecting an area, make a clean circular motion around the site and from the area and move outwardly. Make sure the place is dry and do not palpate again. If needed to palpated, make sure the area is re-cleaned before the venipuncture is carried out again.

10. Request the patient to make a clenched hand; maintain a strategic distance from "siphoning the clench hand." Grasp the patient's arm immovably, utilizing your thumb to draw the skin rigid and anchor the vein. Quickly embed the needle through the skin into the lumen of the vein. The needle should shape a 15-30-degree point with the arm surface.

11. At the point when the last tube is filling, remove the tourniquet.

12. Remove the needle from the patient's arm utilizing a quick in reverse movement.

13. Place wool promptly on the cut site. Apply and hold sufficient strain to maintain a strategic distance from the hematoma. Hold pressure for 1-2 minutes, tape a new piece of bandage or Band-Aid to the cut site.

14. Discard used materials/supplies in assigned holders.

Heel stick Procedure (for infants)

1. Pre-warming the heel (42° C for 3 to 5 minutes) is critical to build the progression of blood for assortment.

2. Wash your hands, and put gloves on. Clean the site to be penetrated with a spirit. Dry the cleaned region with a dry bandage cushion.

3. Hold the infant's foot solidly to evade abrupt development.

4. Utilizing a sterile blood security lancet, cut the heel's side in the fitting districts that appeared previously. Cut with the goal that a drop of blood can gush and not run along the lines. So, make a clean cut across the lines.

5. Wipe away the principal drop of blood with a piece of perfect, dry cotton dressing. Since infants do not frequently drain quickly, utilize delicate strain to create an adjusted drop of blood. Try not to use excessive pressing factors since the blood may get weakened with tissue liquid.

6. Fill in the required micro trainer(s) as demanded.

7. When completed, hoist the heel, place a piece of spotless, dry cotton on the cut site, and hold it set up until the draining has stopped. Apply tape or Band-Aid to the place if necessary.

8. Make sure to discard the lancet in the fitting sharps compartment. Discard used materials in proper waste containers.

9. Disgrace your gloves and wash your hands.

Fingerstick Procedure

1. Follow steps (one) through (six) of the system for venipuncture as laid out above.

2. The best areas for fingersticks are the third (center) and fourth (ring) fingers of the non-predominant hand. Try not to utilize the tip of the finger or the focal point of the finger. Keep a distance from the finger's tip where there is a less delicate tissue, where vessels and nerves are found, and where the bone is nearer to the surface. The second (pointer) will, in general, have thicker, callused skin.
   The fifth finger will, in general, have less delicate tissue overlying the bone. Try not to penetrate a finger that is cold or cyanotic, swollen, scarred, or covered with a rash.

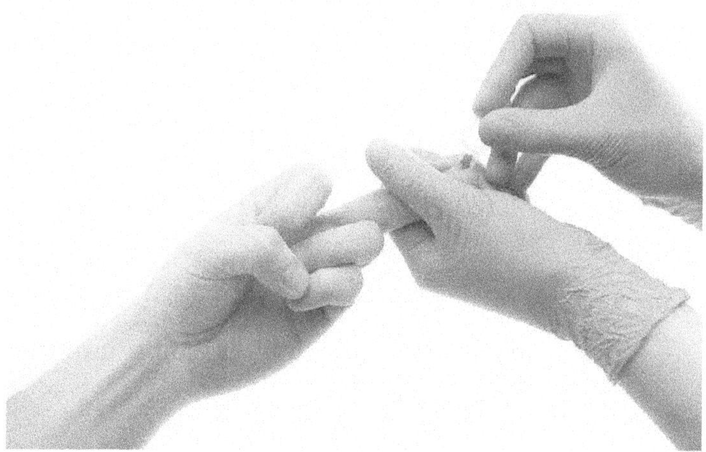

3. When a site is chosen, put on gloves, and cleanse the chose cut zone.

4. Back rub the finger toward the marked site preceding the cut.

5. Utilizing a sterile safety lancet, make a skin cut simply off the focal point of the finger cushion. The cut ought to be made opposite to the edges of the unique mark, so the drop of blood doesn't run down the edges.

6. Clean off the primary drop of blood, which will, in general, contain overabundance tissue liquid.

7. Gentle pressure on the finger, and collect drops of blood into the collection tube/device. "Milking" may compress tissue fluid into the drop of blood - avoid excessive force.

8. Cover, twist, and alter the collection device to mix the blood.

9. Politely instruct the patient to hold a small bandage pad over the puncture position for some minutes to stop blood from flowing.

10. Discard used materials/supplies in the right waste bin or container.

11. Give the right labelling to the patient's tubes at the bedside.

A final note on Methods to Prevent hemolysis (which can meddle with numerous tests):

- Blend all tubes with anticoagulant added substances tenderly (vigorous shaking can cause hemolysis) 5-10 times.
- Try not to draw blood from a hematoma; select another draw area.
- While utilizing suctioning, try not to step the unclogged back too powerfully.
- Ensure the venipuncture site is dry before blood withdrawal.
- Keep away from an examining, awful venipuncture.
- Maintain a strategic distance from delayed tourniquet application (close to 2 minutes; under 1 moment is ideal).
- Abstain from rubbing, crushing, or testing a site.
- Dodge over the top clench, hand gripping.
- In the event that the bloodstream into the tube eases back, change the needle position to stay in the focal point of the lumen.

1.4 Urine Specimen Collection and Processing

Urine collection is in two stages, and they are direct collection by the patient and via the use of a catheter. Whichever way, it is necessary for anyone involved to observe the **clean-catch midstream specimen.** This applies to urine collection so that all bacteria and some other contaminants are prevented from getting into the urine sample.

Collect urine sample directly:

1. Give the patient a urine container in order to collect the urine sample, following the "*clean-catch midstream* – that is, the patient does not contain the first stream of urine and the last stream.

2. Prepare a label with the patient's details on it. And this can be medical records, name, date of birth. Avoid incorrect labeling, make sure the details are input in the patient's presence to avoid any complications afterwards.

3. Collection of data varies according to hospital as well as facility policies. Copy the lab request form and attach it to the specimen.

4. Make sure you wear gloves, and perform all the hygienic procedures while handling the specimen.

5. Explain to the patient why there is a need to collect his urine, and provide with the container, urinal, or bedpan to receive it.

Collect urine sample using a catheter

1. Set the catheter 30 minutes before collecting the specimen. This way, the urine can be collected in the bladder.

2. Clamp the tube below the point of collecting the sample.

3. Clean the sampling port with alcohol if the drainage tube has one.

4. Insert a syringe to take the required sample at a 90-degree angle.

5. Unclamp the tube after collecting the sample.

6. Properly store the sample in a container for further testing.

Tips to perform clean-catch midstream specimen

Before doing anything else, clean the urinary meatus and its surrounding tissue. This is one of the procedures to collect an uncontaminated urine sample. Instruct your patient to start the stream, and collect the piece in the middle of the steam.

Instruct a male patient to clean the tip of his penis with soap and water or with the povidone-iodine solution or chloroprene. This is necessary to make the site free of contaminants. Then, the patient starts the stream and collects the sample in the middle of the steam—the male patient stream without stopping before taking the sample in the middle of the stream.

Instruct the female patient to clean her genital areas with soap and water. Also, with disposable wipes, instruct her to wipe down with soaked povidone-iodine solution or chloroprene. Instruct her to wipe down first, then one side, and the middle of labial folds, vulva, and urinary meatus. In other to avoid fecal contamination, wiping from front to back needs to be the first option. Instruct her to start the stream, and begin the specimen collection in the middle of the stream. If the outside of the container is wet, clean it up and wipe it dry.

1.5 Stool Specimen Collection and Processing

A clean technique must be the critical goal of stool specimen collection since this prevents inappropriate treatment and improves results as well. Although some patient can easily collect their sample themselves, you must explain the significance of each process and how they can refrain from contaminating the specimen. All in all, good hygiene should be highly emphasized even if the patient is collecting the sample by him/herself.

Another case is the presence of urine. When urine is present in the sample, the stool can still be processed in the laboratory by using various techniques to separate the urine's stool.

Summary of the equipment needed:

- The disposable receiver or bedpan
- Non-sterile gloves
- Apron
- Specimen bag
- Pulp tray
- Sterile specimen pot with an integral spoon

Obtaining a stool sample

1. Ensure privacy and dignity are well observed, as this procedure may be embarrassing to patients.

2. Clean the contacted areas (no risk of cross-infection yet) and assemble the equipment.

3. Put on non-sterile gloves and an apron in order to reduce the risk of cross-infection.

4. Ensure to request that the patient passes urine before taking the stool sample – this avoids urine mixing with feces and contaminating the sample.

5. Ask to the patient to defecate into the bedpan, otherwise known as a collector.

6. When the patient is not active, a sample can be extracted from the bed linen, but contamination with urine should definitely be monitored.

7. Enough sample is collected by using the integral spoon in the sample pot to fill around a quarter of the specimen pot. The feces should be either liquid or semi-formed and take on the shape of the container.

8. Seal the covering of the sample-container.

9. Remove all the disposable material and dispose of it right after use.

10. Clean the contacted places with soap and water in order to reduce the risk of cross-infection. Alcohol hand rubs are ineffective against C difficile and should not be used when handling potentially infected stools.

11. Examine the specimen and record the color, consistency, and odor of the stool as part of the clinical assessment.

12. If there is a delay in transportation, specimen.
13. It can be refrigerated but should be processed within 12 hours. It is crucial to review local policy for further information about conveyance and storage if these infections are suspected and the sample should be sent to the laboratory as quickly as possible.

https://labtestsonline.org/articles/laboratory-testing-tips-coping

https://www.britannica.com/science/blood-biochemistry

Chapter 2: Hematological Test

2.1 Complete Blood Count CBC

This is a set of medical tests and findings that give insight into the amount of blood present in a patient. Notably, it indicates the count of the white & red blood cells, platelets, the concentration of hemoglobin, and the hematocrit. The test is carried out on a regular basis by comparing the results with standard reference ranges, which vary with sex, age, and some other values.

There are many means of counting the blood, and among them is the laboratory approach with the equipment known as the automated hematology analyzer. This automated hematology analyzer compared the blood via collation via sizes and structure. Furthermore, the blood sample concentration is known in the aspect of the red blood cells and hemoglobin.

Why Get Tested?

Testing for CBC is useful to know the general blood count, see the nature or causes of some disease, monitor and diagnose various conditions, especially those that affect blood cells. They include anemia, infection, inflammation.

When to Test?

Often, a test is carried out on a patient when signs and symptoms related to a blood condition are noticed and when there is a need to know general blood counts and monitor the level of disease.

What is Being Tested?

There are main cells that the CBC evaluates, and they are:

1. **Red Blood Cells**

The red blood cells have 120 days lifespan. The cell is produced in the bone marrow and matures in the body until the lifespan is reached. Additionally, it contains hemoglobin, and this is the element that transports oxygen through the body.

2. **White Blood Cells**

The blood cells are a defensive cell that fights against diseases. And it is found in the blood, the lymphatic system, and the tissues. It protects against infections, inflammation, and allergic reactions.

3. **Platelets**

They are significant for blood clotting. They are found as tiny particles in the blood cells. Platelets also release chemical changes that initiate the clumping of additional platelets.

What is included in a CBC?

A CBC is regularly performed utilizing an instrument that estimates different boundaries, including cell counts and the actual highlights of a portion of the cells. A standard CBC incorporates:

Red platelet (RBC) tests:

- Red platelet (RBC) count checks the real number of red platelets in your blood test.
- Hemoglobin quantifies the aggregate sum of the oxygen-conveying protein in the blood, which for the most part, mirrors the number of red platelets in the blood.

- Hematocrit quantifies the level of absolute blood volume that comprises red platelets.

- Red platelet files give data on the actual highlights of the RBCs:

  Mean corpuscular volume (MCV) is an estimation of the typical size of your red platelets.

  Mean corpuscular hemoglobin (MCH) is a determined estimation of the standard measure of hemoglobin inside your red platelets.

  Mean corpuscular hemoglobin fixation (MCHC) is a determined estimation of the normal centralization of hemoglobin inside your red platelets.

  Red cell dissemination width (RDW) estimates the variety in the size of red blood cells.

The CBC may likewise incorporate reticulocyte count, which estimates the check or level of recently delivered fresh red blood in the blood test.

White platelet (WBC) tests:

White platelet (WBC) tally is a check of the complete number of white platelets in your blood test.

White platelet differential might be incorporated as a CBC component or might be done in development if the WBC count is maximal or minimal(high or low). The WBC differential distinguishes and checks the quantity of the five kinds of white platelets present (neutrophils, lymphocytes, monocytes, eosinophils, and basophils). The individual components can be accounted for as an outright count or potentially as a level of aggregate.

Platelet tests:

- The platelet test is the number of platelets in the blood.

- Mean platelet volume (MPV) might be accounted for with a CBC. It is an estimation of the average size of platelets.

- Platelets reflect how uniform they are in size. Platelet conveyance width (PDW) may likewise be accounted for.

CBC results revealed outside the setup reference spans may demonstrate at least one infection or condition. Different tests are performed on a regular basis in order to help decide the reason for unusual outcomes. A blood smear will normally be analyzed utilizing a magnifying lens. A prepared lab expert will assess the appearance and actual highlights of the platelets, for example, size, shape, and shading while taking note of any anomalies that might be available. This data gives the medical services extra specialist pieces of information concerning the reason for strange CBC results.

2.2 Test for Anemia

Iron-lack deficiency is a typical weakness that happens in the event that patients need more iron in their body. Individuals with gentle or moderate iron-lack weakness might not have any signs or indications. More iron-inadequacy severe deficiency may cause weariness or sluggishness, or chest torment.

In the event that a caring physician determined that a patient has iron-insufficiency sickliness, the therapy will rely upon the reason as well as seriousness of the condition. The primary care as a physician may suggest smart dieting changes, iron enhancements, intravenous iron treatment for gentle to direct iron-lack weakness, or red platelet bonding for iron-inadequacy severe frailty.

You may have to address the reason for iron insufficiency, for example, any fundamental dying. If undiscovered or untreated, iron-insufficiency pallor might cause genuine confusion, including a cardiovascular breakdown and improvement delays in kids.

Tips for treatment

Iron treatment, or intravenous (IV) iron. This is used to convey iron through a vein to expand iron levels in the blood. One advantage of IV iron is that it frequently takes just one or a couple of meetings to renew the measure of iron in the body. Individuals with iron-lack severe frailty or who are affected by constant conditions such as kidney infection or celiac illness, might be bound to get IV iron. They may encounter spewing, cerebral pain, or opposite results after the IV iron. However, these typically disappear inside a day or two.

Red platelet bonding. These might be utilized for individuals with iron-inadequacy severe frailty to rapidly expand the measure of red platelets and iron in the blood. The PCP may suggest this if they have genuine entanglements of iron-inadequacy frailty, for example, chest torment.

A. Homoglobin Toot

The hemoglobin test measures the level of hemoglobin in the blood. As described, this is the element that carries blood around the body. A low hemoglobin level means low red blood cells -anemia. Anemia has various symptoms as well as signs, which include vitamin deficiency, bleeding, and chronic diseases. If the hemoglobin level is higher than usual, it also shows an abnormality, which may be due to smoking and dehydration, among many others.

Why hemoglobin test?

A hemoglobin test is mandatory to check for overall health performance. If a patient shows symptoms related to blood level, ah emoglobin count can be done to prevent how well oxygen and other elements are transported through the body systems.

Also, a hemoglobin test is viable when a patient experiences weakness, fatigue, shortness, and dizziness. All these might be due to a shortage of blood that will circulate the necessary nutrients. And these signs may likewise indicate anemia or **polycythemia vera.**

A hemoglobin test can be used to monitor the level of performance after running through an anemia or polycythemia diagnosis.

What hemoglobin test is

For an adult, the sample of blood can be taken by pricking the finger or collecting via a needle. Also, an infant's blood sample can be taken by pricking the heel.

On the normal range, the hemoglobin ranges from:

- 12.0 - 15.5 grams/deciliter **(Women)**
- 13.5 - 17.5 grams/deciliter **(Men)**

However, normal hemoglobin ranges differ in children, and each practitioner can decide on a normal range for him/herself.

Some of the condition that contributes to low hemoglobin level are the following:

- Bleeding
- Kidney disease
- Liver disease
- Hypothyroidism
- Folate deficiency
- Leukemia or other blood cancer

- Iron deficiency
- Liver disease

In case of high hemoglobin level, it can be due to:

- Smoking
- Burns
- Lung disease
- Dehydration
- Excessive vomiting
- Living in high places

What is the Hematocrit?

An automated machine is used to measure the hematocrit (HCT). Hematocrit is the percentage of the blood that contains red blood cells. Another alternative is centrifugation to determine the level of hematocrit; then, the amount of red blood cell to the total level of blood can be measured – thus measuring the hematocrit.

Normal ranges of hematocrit based on age differences

Age	Hematocrit Percentage
Adult Women	38% to 46%
Adult Males	42% to 52%
10 Years Old	36% to 40%
1 Year Old	29% to 41%
3 Months Old	30% to 36%
1 Month Old	37% to 49%
1 Week Old	47% to 65%
Newborn	55% to 68%

Red blood cell indices and Calculation

Red blood cell indices have two central values. First, they are sued to differentiate anemias and are used as quality control checkers on various lab testing.

The necessary means of red blood cells indices are:

- Mean cell hemoglobin concentration (MCHC)
- Mean cell hemoglobin (MCH)
- Mean cell volume (MCV)

Parameters	**Measurements**	**Units**
Mean cell hemoglobin concentration	This is the mean concentration of hemoglobin in red blood cell volume	g/dL
Mean cell volume	The red blood cell average volume	fL or 10^{-15} Liter
Mean cell hemoglobin	The mean weight of the hemoglobin in the red blood cell	pg or 10^{-12} grams

These boundaries distinguish attributes of the red cells that are flowing when the specimen was gathered. The table above sums up the three limits to incorporate definition, announcing units, and units for every boundary count.

MCV alludes to the standard size of the RBCs establishing the example. Should a combination of cell populaces be available, the red cells' measures will be found the median value. Announcing units is femtoliters (fL). One femtoliter is 10-15 L. Reference span for grown-ups usually is 80 - 100 fL.

Mean cell hemoglobin (MCH) alludes to the usual load of hemoglobin in the RBCs in the example. Should a combination of cell populaces be available, limitations of the assessed cells will be found the median value of. Announcing units is picograms (pg). One picogram is 10 - 12 grams. The reference span for grown-ups is commonly 26 - 32 pg.

Mean cell hemoglobin fixation (MCHC) alludes to the normal centralization of hemoglobin in the RBCs contained inside the example. Should a combination of cell populaces be available, the hemoglobin focus inside the assessed cells will be found the median value of. Revealing units is g/dL. The reference stretch for grown-ups usually is 32 - 36 g/dL.

2.3 Advanced Test for Anemia

Approach to Peripheral Blood Smear

The basic idea of the peripheral blood smear is examining a blood sample under the microscope to check the different blood count and their shapes. All the blood cells (white blood cells, red blood cells, platelets, and others) have specific forms as well as flow. The peripheral blood smear gives a straightforward interpretation of any hematological problems and aims for reasonable blood investigation. The results of the procedure are often processed between 24 to 36 hours.

Peripheral blood smear gives a direct result of the blood information, and the data can include the following:

- Analyze a scope of inadequacies, illnesses, and during chemo/radiation treatment
- It recognizes different sorts of white platelets
- In the assessment for hemoglobin variations
- It analyzes if red platelets, white platelets, and platelets are ordinary in appearance and number
- Shows their overall rates in the blood

- Shows if Malaria/Filaria is present in the patient

Interpreting Peripheral Blood Smear

A blood smear is viewed as ordinary when the blood contains an adequate number of cells and a typical appearance. A blood smear is considered irregular when there's a variation from the norm in the size, shape, shading, or number of cells in your blood. Uneven outcomes may shift contingent upon the sort of platelet influenced.

Red blood problems include:

- iron-deficiency, a situation where the body does not create enough red blood cell because of iron insufficiency

- sickle cell iron deficiency, an acquired illness that occurs when red platelets have an unusual bow shape

- hemolytic uremic disorder, which is generally set off by a disease in the stomach related framework

- polycythemia rubra vera, a problem that happens when the body produces an extreme number of red platelets

Issues identified with white platelets include:

- Chronic leukemia, a sort of blood malignancy
- Lymphoma, a type of disease that influences the invulnerable framework
- HIV, an infection that taints white platelets
- Hepatitis C infection disease
- Parasitic diseases, for example, pinworm
- Contagious diseases, for example, candidiasis
- Other lymphoproliferative illnesses, including different myeloma

Problems influencing platelets include:

- Myeloproliferative issues, issues that cause platelets to fill unusual in the bone marrow
- Thrombocytopenia, which happens when the quantity of platelets is deficient because of contamination or other sicknesses

A blood smear can likewise show different conditions, including:

- Liver illness
- Kidney illness
- Hypothyroidism

Regular and irregular values can shift among labs since some utilize various instruments or strategies to dissect the blood test. You should consistently examine your outcomes in more detail with your superiors. They must have the option to advise you if you need further testing.

Serum Iron

This is the procedure that measures the circulating iron and the serum. That is the **transferrin and the ferritin.** This approach is an advanced test for anemia, and it is performed clinically when there are symptoms that either show a lack of iron or the presence of anemia in a patient.

Average values for serum iron

Serum Iron	Values
Women	50 to 170 ug/dL
Men	65 to 176 ug/dL
Children	50 to 120 ug/dL
Newborns	100 to 250 ug/dL

- **TIBC:** 240 - 450 ug/dL
- **Transferrin saturation:** 20 - 50 %

Schilling Test

The test is used for patients with vitamin B_{12} deficiency. The procedure is based on how a patient can absorb vitamin B12. And it occurs in two stages.

Stage 1

The patient must receive radiolabeled nutrient B12 orally, and after one hour, the patient is given an intramuscular (IM) portion of unlabeled nutrient B12. The infusion is given to guarantee that none of the radioactive B12 binds to any nutrient B12 exhausted tissues, for instance, the liver.
A 24-hour urine sample screens the ingestion and the discharge.

In the event that stage 1 is strange, step 2 might be done 3 to 7 days after.
Stage 2

In the event that the last stage gives an uncommon outcome, stage 2 should be possible to evaluate whether there is a lack of inborn factor Stage 1 is performed again, alongside an oral portion of inherent factor. A 24-hour urine assortment is done to survey the degree of nutrient B12.

Signs

Patients showing signs and symptoms of cobalamin go through this test. The most well-known highlights of nutrient B12 inadequacy incorporate severe macrocytic frailty and variable neurologic anomalies, for example, rearranging stride, with no improvement saw upon the organization of folic corrosive.

2.4 Test for Blood Coagulation

Clotting is essential for life survival, especially in making the best of cuts and reducing the aftermath of blood loss. Notwithstanding, blood moving through the body must not clot. If something like this happens, it may travel to the heart, liver, or other organs and block the smooth flow of the blood, which in turn leads to heart attack, stroke, or death.

The main goal of this test is to know how fast patient blood clots. And this will give useful insights into the danger of excessive blood loss as well as chances to suffer from blood clotting in the body.

Types of coagulation test

S/N	Coagulation Test	Measurements
1.	Factor V assay	The test measures one of the factor (Factor V) which aids blood clotting. If it is low, that might be an indication of liver disease.
2.	Complete blood count	This gives insight into how well the blood or platelets are in blood clotting. It is a smooth way to know the capability of patient blood to clot.
3.	Fibrinogen Level	Fibrinogen test measures the amount of fibrinogen. Since the level produces it, abnormal results can show **hemorrhage,**

		fibrinolysis, and placental abruption.
4.	Platelet Count	Platelet helps in blood clotting. The abnormal level of platelet cells may be due to excessive bleeding, chemotherapy, or medication. Additionally, a high abnormality level of platelet may be due to **anemia, thrombocythemia, and leukemia**.
5.	Prothrombin Time (PT-INR)	The prothrombin measures how the patient blood clot in actions of time. The liver produces this blood protein component. On the normal range, it takes about 25 to 30 seconds to clot. However, this may vary if the patient

		takes blood thinners. And the time also varies due to **hemophilia, liver disease, and malabsorption**.
6.	Thrombin Time	Throbbing Time measures how fibrinogen in the blood is working in respect of blood clotting. Often, abnormality comes from genetic fibrinogen disorder, blood cancer, liver disease, and even medications.
7.	Bleeding Time	This test examines how rapidly little veins in the skin close up and quit dying. It's performed uniquely in contrast to the previous blood tests. A pulse sleeve will be put on the patient's upper arm and swelled. The medical care

		supplier will make several little cuts on the patient's lower arm. The cuts will not be deep and will, for the most part, feel like scratches. The medical care supplier will eliminate the sleeve when it is flattened and momentarily place blotching paper on the cuts at regular intervals until draining stops. Draining ordinarily endures between 1 to 9 minutes. The test is viewed as protected and common side effects.

2.5 Blood Grouping and Typing

The main classification of blood is due to the presence or absence of antibiotics and inherited antigenic substances (which can be proteins, carbohydrates, glycoproteins, and glycolipids) from the parent. Most of the time, these antigens are located on the surface of the red blood cells, which play many roles in blood grouping and typing.

Blood group systems include **ABO blood group system, Eh blood group system, ABO, and Eh distribution by country.**

Significances of blood group systems include "*blood transfusion, hemolytic disease of the newborn, blood products, red blood cell compatibility, plasma compatibility, and universal donors & universal recipients.*

	Group A	**Group B**	**Group AB**	**Group O**
Red Blood Cell Type	A	B	AB	O
Antibiotics in Plasma	Anti-B	Anti-A	None	Anti-A and Anti-B
Antigens in Red Blood Cell	An antigen	B antigen	A and B antigens	None

https://www.nlm.nih.gov/medlineplus/ency/article/003423.htm

http://www.nhs.uk/chq/Pages/1018.aspx?CategoryID=69&SubCategoryID=693

Chapter 3: Cardiac Enzymes Used in Myocardial

Cardiac enzymes are biomarkers that are used to diagnose heart conditions and functions. They are useful in the primary stage of predicting or diagnosing heart diseases. Most of the early markers are identified enzymes, and they are not always enzymes. These enzymes include myoglobin, troponin, and creatine kinase. They are released into the blood whenever myocardial necrosis occurs.

Myoglobin

Myoglobin is similar to hemoglobin in structure, although it is found in muscle tissues, unlike hemoglobin. It binds to iron as well as oxygen. Myoglobin is not a direct cardiac enzyme. However, it is used in conjunction with cardiac enzymes in order to carryout myocardial tests.

Myoglobin is released when there is damage to the muscle tissues, and this includes myocardial necrosis. Myoglobin is more suitable for various tests because results can easily be seen after 30 minutes of administration, unlike troponin and creatine kinase. However, the measurements of skeletal muscle with myoglobin are nonspecific for MIs.

Myoglobin aids the process of measuring the amount of muscle damage but cannot give the exact location of the tissue damage. Elevate myoglobin has low specificity for acute myocardial infarction (AMI), and thus CK-MB, cardiac troponin, ECG. And to make the diagnosis more significant, clinical signs should be taken into account.

The values of myoglobin are 25 - 200 U/L. It elevates 4 to 6 hours after an acute MI, peaks in 18 to 24 hours, and returns to normal within 3 to 4 days.

Troponin

Troponin is a cardiac enzyme. It is in two forms – troponin I and troponin T. It is released into the circulation about 3 and 4 following myocardial infarction, and it is detectable for about 10 days. This long circulation makes it viable for late MI diagnosis, but it is not easy at all to detect re-infarction. Troponin is integral in muscle contraction, including skeletal muscle and cardiac muscle, but not smooth muscle. The measurements of troponin I and troponin T are used extensively in the sizes and management of myocardial infarction and acute coronary syndrome.

Troponin is significant in measuring instability in angina and myocardial infarction (heart attack) by monitoring patient blood, especially those with chest pain as well as auto coronary syndrome.

The enzymes are administered in 2-4 hours and peak within 10-24 hours of MI. It then drops within 1-2 weeks. The value of troponin is < 0.01 ng/ml.

Creatine Phosphokinase or Creatine Kinase

Creatine Phosphokinase is explicitly used on patients with chest pain, although troponin has covered more of the advantages. Typical Creatine Phosphokinase values are between 60 and 400 IU/L. Creatine Phosphokinase may be high in patients with health and specific diseases. In addition, an excess increase of creatine kinase is another reason for high Creatine Phosphokinase.

High Creatine Phosphokinase may indicate damage to CK-rich tissue such as rhabdomyolysis, myocardial infarction, myositis, and myocarditis.

Creatine Phosphokinase has three isomers, which include CK-MB, CK-BB, CK-MM.

CK MB is found in the skeletal and cardiac muscle, CK-BB is located in the brain tissue, and the isomer CK-MM is also found in the skeletal and cardiac muscle.

It elevates 4 to 6 hours after an acute MI, peaks in 18 to 24 hours, and returns to normal within 3 to 4 days.

Creatine Phosphokinase cannot be used for late diagnosis, as it has a short duration of increase.

Lactase dehydrogenase

This enzyme is significant in the conversion of lactic acid to pyruvic acid, and this is the primary step in glycolysis. Lactase dehydrogenase increases if there is tissue damage and thus can be used to measure the level of a cardiac condition. There are five isomers of LDH (LDH1, LDH2, LDH3, LDH4, and LDH5). LD1 is found in the heart, red blood cells, and kidneys. And these are the two central which contribute to myocardial and its diagnosis.

The typical values 140 - 280 U/L, and the total LDH rises between 2 - 5 days after an MI. The elevated level lasts for 10 days.

The amount and level of LDH vary; even if the total value is within the normal range, the isozymes level may be altered.

And this demands that the level ratio of the various isozymes is checked.

	LDH-1	LDH-2
Values	17.5% - 28.3%	30.4% - 36.4%

From the table above, LDH-2 is higher than LDH-1. When the acute MI is performed, the level of LDH-2 does not change, but the level of LDH-1 rises. This condition is defined as **flipped state**. And it appears 12 - 24 hours after an MI.

Serum Glutamine Oxaloacetate Transaminase

SGOT is a pyridoxal phosphate enzyme, and it catalyzes the reversible transfer of an alpha-amino group between aspartate and glutamate. The enzymes are found in the liver, heart: skeletal muscle, kidneys, red blood cells, and brain.

It has two isoenzymes, and they are located in the eukaryotes. The SGOT1/cAST is situated in the red blood cells and heart. It is a cytosolic isoenzyme. Also, the SGOT2/mAST is located in the liver— and it is a mitochondria isoenzyme.

SGOT spikes in 8 to 12 hours after infarction, and it reaches a peak at 24 - 48 hours after infarction. The standard value is 5 - 50 IU/L.

It is majorly used as conjunction enzymes with other enzymes. It is not particularly indicative of MI as serum levels of SGOT can increase due to liver and pancreatic disease.

The pattern of enzyme levels during MI

Cardiac troponins T and I have the highest sensitivity and specifications for diagnosing acute myocardial infarction, and they remain the preferred markers for the condition.

Patients with negative heart biomarkers inside six hours of the beginning of indications that are steady with ACS should have biomarkers premeasured in the time of twelve hours after the beginning of side effects.

Peak circling enzyme levels will, in general, happen prior and are frequently higher after effective thrombolytic treatment.

Cardiovascular troponin I and T have myoglobin and creatine kinase-MB as the favored markers of myocardial injury. Notwithstanding, vulnerabilities, and questions stay on the estimation of high-affectability cardiovascular troponin tests, including their best clinical use.

Troponin is a protein delivered from myocytes when irreversible myocardial harm happens. It is profoundly explicit to heart tissue and precisely determined myocardial localized necrosis to have a background marked by ischemic agony or ECG changes reflecting ischemia. Cardiovascular troponin level is subject to infarct size, along these lines giving a marker to the anticipation following an infarction.

New high-affectability cardiovascular troponin tests have been built up that can gauge troponin values at much lower levels. With the utilization of these high-affectability examinations, more patients with shaky angina will be named having non-ST-elevation myocardial dead tissue. These tests may, in this way, characterize a risky patient populace and may prompt more suitable treatment and improved results in these patients.

Heart troponins T and I are profoundly delicate and explicit for cardiovascular harm. Troponin I and T are of equivalent clinical worth.

Serum levels increment inside 3-12 hours from the beginning of chest pain, peak at 24-48 hours, and return baseline more than 5-14 days.

Troponin levels may not be distinguishable for six hours after the beginning of myocardial cell injury. The early marker for dead myocardial tissue is myoglobin.

Troponin levels should be estimated at the introduction and again 10-12 hours after the beginning of indications. When there is a vulnerability concerning the hour of side effect beginning, troponin should be estimated at twelve hours after the introduction.

The chances of death from an ACS are straightforwardly identified with troponin level, and patients with no perceivable troponins have a decent transient guess.

Raised troponin levels can happen in patients without an ACS and are related to unfriendly results in several other clinical circumstances, including congestive cardiovascular breakdown, sepsis, intense pulmonary embolism, and chronic kidney illness. Other cardiovascular causes incorporate myocarditis as well as aortic dissection.

3.1 Lipid Profile

Lipids play a role in various stages in humans. From the function of producing hormones, absorption of nutrients, and also digestion. The lipid profile breakdown the levels of different lipids that are in the body. This test detects or reflects the stories of two essential lipids — cholesterol and triglyceride; and three lipoproteins.

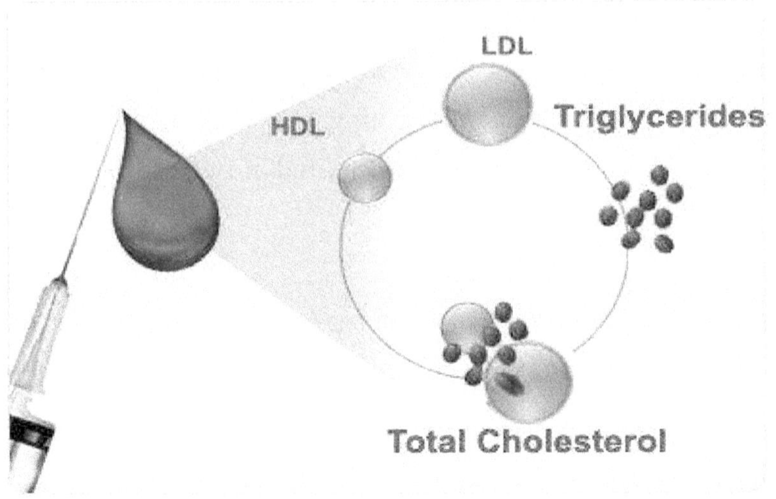

Low-density lipoprotein:

Low-density lipoprotein is also called "bad fat"; it transports cholesterol from the liver to various parts of the body. Low-density lipoprotein has a good interaction with high-density lipoprotein.

High-density lipoprotein:

High-density lipoprotein transports cholesterol from the tissues around the body to the liver (where it is produced). This concept prevents excess cholesterol blood levels. The high-density lipoprotein cleans off cholesterol from the walls of blood vessels and flushes it out through flows of blood, and this prevents atherosclerotic narrowing of blood vessels.

When a patient is diagnosed with a high level of (high-density lipoprotein), it is a sign of good health unless it is biased with a disease or some other conditions.

Very low-density lipoprotein (VLDL):

Unlike high-density and low-density lipoprotein, very low-density lipoprotein serves as the body's internal transportation system for lipids. And also, it doesn't transport only cholesterol; it also transports triglycerides within the body.

Triglycerides:

Body fats are converted and stored in triglycerides, and these fats are broken down when the lipids in the body are needed to supply energy to various metabolic stages. A high triglyceride level shows any of the following conditions: hypothyroidism, myocardial infarction, nephrotic syndrome, liver disease, metabolic disorders, atherosclerosis, pancreatitis as well as toxemia.

Total Cholesterol

Cholesterol has various clinical functions, aside from the side effects in cardiovascular conditions.

- Cellular, it forms the integral parts of the cell wall and plays a vital role in regulating substances in the cellular field. Additionally, it plays the part of crucial role in the production of steroid hormones in the body. It also activates vitamin D that is formed from exposure to the sun.

The human body will be low in cholesterol due to anemia, malignancies, liver insufficiency, depression, and malnutrition. Also, an increase in cholesterol level is a factor of hypothyroidism, atherosclerosis, diabetes, and pregnancy.

THE Cholesterol HDL ratio shows the amount of HDL in the total cholesterol. Total cholesterol includes the fat contained in LDL, HDL, and triglycerides. If the balance is high, there is an increased risk of developing atherosclerotic. And it can be calculated by dividing the total cholesterol level by HDL level.

https://doi.org/10.1146%2Fannurev-pathmechdis-012418-012827

http://emedicine.medscape.com/article/811905-overview

Chapter 4: Serum Electrolytes

Electrolytes are the various ions that contribute to the regulation of several functions in the body, mostly involved in the cations and anions interactions. The level of these ions must be the same to have good results in all areas regarding the serum electrolytes. And this includes the blood and the other regions. Electrolytes are applicable in the transfer of information across the nerves and also aid proper muscle contraction and relaxation.

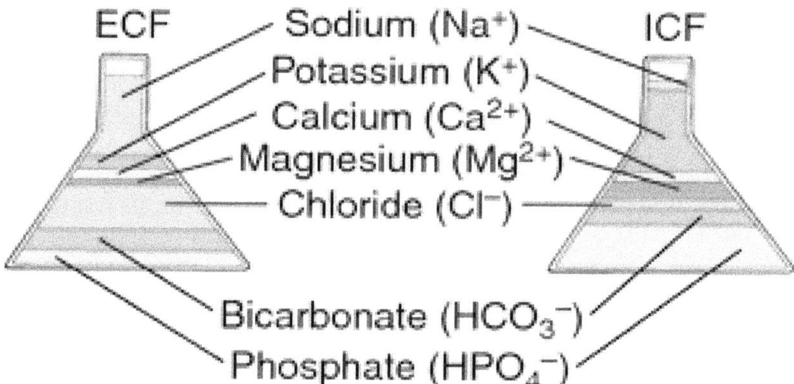

- In children: the leading cause of dehydration and electrolyte imbalance include acute gastroenteritis. And this condition is orally treated by supplying water to hydrate.

- In adults: less caring altitude for dehydration and thirst often leads to an elevated risk of dehydration and electrolyte imbalance. And it is majorly treated with current hydration.

Electrolyte Imbalance

Electrolyte imbalance simply means inequality in the levels of the electrolytes that are flowing through the body. Electrolytes such as calcium are not alone; they are balanced with other charges (cations and anions). When the level of these charges is not equal, it might reduce the chance of disease. Functions of electrolytes include water balance, regulating the body's base pH levels, and moving nutrients and waste products from the body.

Checking for electrolyte imbalance can be the right approach to detect illness lying-in patients. An electrolyte imbalance understands a sickness that is majorly due to homeostasis balance. Ways to access the body for balanced electrolytes is by physical examination. ECGs, serum electrolytes levels, and other signs portray by the patient.

A thorough study of the electrolytic system can mostly give you a direct link to the primary electrolyte lacking in the body. An example is the case of **hypocalcemia. A patient** that shows signs such as confusion may have hypocalcemia.
Some of the signs which indicate electrolyte imbalance include:

- Fever
- Confusion
- Atrial fibrillation
- Abdominal pain
- Edema
- Rales
- Dyspnoea
- Fever
- Systemic deterioration

What Causes an Electrolyte Imbalance

Dehydration is a significant factor that is used to indicate electrolyte imbalance. Many determinants indicate dehydration, and one of them is a dry mouth. However, dry mouth is an uncertain sign to pinpoint dehydration as it is not clinically sufficient to indicate dehydration.

When the body is over-hydrated, the body filtering system cannot function as it should be. And this impairs the electrolyte in the body. The inner system also contributes to balanced or unbalanced electrolytes.

When actions like severe burns, vomiting, diarrhea, and excessive sweating occurs, it disrupts the internal balance system. In other terms, when the body has more than usual water in comparison to the ions in the body, this contributes to unbalanced electrolytes.

Electrolyte Imbalance Risk Factors

Most of the conditions that can show electrolyte imbalance are not significantly sure to compare to situations such as *diabetes, hypertension, and use of diuretics.* Diabetes and hypertension contribute to electrolyte imbalance, but not as diuretics. Also, patients with diabetes conditions combined with diuretics are at a more considerable risk of electrolyte imbalance than others in this stage. For example, a patient who uses both thiazides and benzodiazepines is associated with a higher risk of hyponatremia. Patients with this condition are at higher risk of mortality. In general, electrolyte Imbalance can be mild and severe in different cases. Also, ACE inhibitors, potassium, and calcium supplements with some hormones can lead to electrolyte imbalances.

Diagnosing an Electrolyte Imbalance

Several approaches are applicable in testing electrolyte imbalance, and they all have their side effects alongside the significances.

- **The Anion Gap Blood Test**: this test analyses the level of blood acid, and it can be used to indicate an electrolyte imbalance. Likewise, it is a suitable means of balancing the blood pH.

- **Carbon Dioxide Blood Tests:** he is used to testing the level of CO_2 in the blood. The CO_2 in the blood is called bicarbonates.

- **Chloride test**: measures the amount of chlorine in the blood.

- **Sodium test**: measures the level of sodium in the blood.

4.1 The Important Serum Electrolyte

Sodium

The kidney regulates the parameter of the blood sodium with hormones such as aldosterone and atrial natriuretic peptide. And sodium takes a larger part of the percentage. Sodium alone has 95% of the electrolytes present in the extracellular fluid. Sodium is essential in transportation and plays a role in regulating the osmotic and acid-base balance of the body.

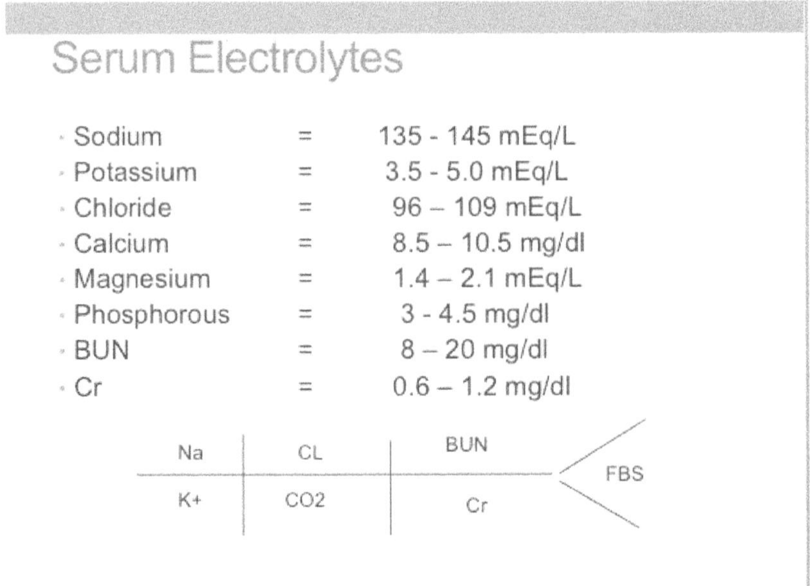

The expected value is 135 - 145mmol/l
Sodium levels increase by decreased water in the body and conditions like impaired thirst mechanism, diabetes insipidus, increased mineralocorticoids, and hyperaldosteronism. Hypernatremia occurs at serum sodium more significant than 145 mEq/L.

High low of sodium is due to increased body fluid, heart failure, ascites, hyperaldosteronism, among others. Hyponatremia occurs when sodium is below 134 mEq/L.

Potassium

Potassium is an intracellular electrolyte, and its level is low in the intercellular plasma. Potassium is critical to normal nerve and muscle function, and it has a narrow reference range. The standard or conventional range is 3.5 to 5.0 mmol/L. Hypokalemia occurs when the potassium level is less than 3.5 mmol/L. Common causes are due to oral intake, increase the renal loss of potassium from outside where the cell it is located. Hypokalemia is caused by muscle weakness ileus and serious cardiac arrhythmias such as ventricular tachycardias.

The cause of increased potassium levels is not known. However, conditions like burns or trauma, renal failure can cause hyperkalemia. This condition occurs when serum potassium is more significant than 5.0 mmol/L. Standard clinical measures that cause high potassium include hypotension, bradycardia, muscle weakness, and ECG changes when T waves peak and P waves flattered.

Magnesium

Magnesium plays a role in transportation, metabolism, and replication in the intercellular cells. The normal range is between 0.70 to 0.95 mmol/L. Magnesium has a strong effect on muscle contractions. Abnormality in the magnesium level can occur with some other electrolyte imbalances; the same reason patients with renal failure must be monitored for magnesium deficiency.

Hypomagnesemia or lack of magnesium has clinical signs, which include confusion, irritability, delirium, and tachycardias. Low magnesium levels cause arrhythmias and need to be corrected immediately. Hypomagnesemia occurs when magnesium is below 0.70.

Hypernatremia is not common, and it is a condition where serum magnesium is higher than the normal range. That is, above 0.95mmol/L. Symptoms include low blood pressure, respiratory depression, cardiac arrest, and poor reflexes.

Calcium

Calcium is an essential element in the body, and it plays a role as some serum calcium control nerve impulses, plays a role in blood clotting and muscle contractions. The normal serum calcium range is between 2.2 to 2.55 mmol/L.

Hypocalcemia, which is low serum calcium is relatively uncommon as the bone acts as a reservoir for this electrolyte. Notwithstanding, various conditions like parathyroid disease, vitamin D deficiency, septic shock, and acute pancreatitis can cause hypocalcemia. Hypocalcemia is seen in hypoparathyroidism or vitamin D deficiency.

Calcium high level in the blood is called Hypercalcemia. And it is due to parathyroid conditions and vitamin D issues. Some of the requirements include nausea, polyuria, mental disturbance, muscular weakness, and vomiting.

Phosphorus

Phosphorus is an electrolyte that is used in various functions all around the body. It is not seen as necessary as other electrolytes; it causes several conditions when it is not maintained at normal levels. The normal serum phosphorus is between 0.8 - 1.3 mmol/L.

Hypophosphatemia is a condition when the phosphorus level in the blood is low—and majorly caused by too much alcohol, deficiency of Vitamin D, and hyperparathyroidism.

Hyperphosphatemia occurs when the level of serum phosphorus is higher than average. A high level of phosphorus does not usually show symptoms, but it can be related to hypocalcemia. The condition can be caused by metabolic acidosis, parathyroid issues, and kidney disease.

Other Blood Values of Electrolytes

This is a summary of the minute electrolytes that play significant importance in the body but are not as relevant as the main ones mentioned above. All in all, the overview of these electrolytes is given below, which includes their values, normal range, and significance.

Electrolyte	**Normal Range**	**Significance**
Zinc	70 - 100 umol/L	Zinc plays an essential role in wound healing, the closing of cut, and cell growth & development
Ammonia	15 - 50 umol/L	Ammonia plays a role in breaking down proteins substances that are metabolized by the liver into urea. And this can increase liver disorders
Copper	70 - 150 ug/dl	Copper has significant roles in the absorption of iron and aids red blood cells incorporation with iron. It is significant in

		several metabolic activities that involve enzymes and proteins
Ceruloplasmin	15 - 60 mg/dl	Ceruloplasmin is a copper carrying proteins. And it is formulated by the liver. It may decrease in a patient affected by a liver disorder
Ferritin	12 - 300 ng/ml in males 12 - 150 ng/ml in females	Ferritin marks the total amount of iron in the body, and it is a carrier of iron.

Pyruvate	300 - 900 ug/dl	Pyruvate is one of the metabolism products (the breakdown of glucose), and it plays a significant role in aerobic respiration.
Urea	1.2 - 3 mmol/l	Urea is a waste of nitrogen and is excreted through the renal system, and it is formed from ammonia in the liver.
Uric acid	0.18 - 0.48 mmol/L	It is formed or accumulated by the degradation of purines. The kidney excretes it; the excess accumulation in the joints can cause gout

Transferrin	65 - 180 ug/dl in males 30 - 170 ug/dl in females	Transferrin aids the transportation of iron from the duodenum to tissues of the body.

https://www.ncbi.nlm.nih.gov/pmc/articles/PMC7226178

https://ui.adsabs.harvard.edu/abs/2009JPS...194...66S

https://en.wikipedia.org/wiki/Energy_%26_Environmental_Science

Chapter 5: Endocrine Function Tests

5.0 Tests for Diabetes

Diabetes is induced by inadequate secretion of insulin (which is responsible for converting glucose into glycogen — the way to store sugar). When the level of blood sugar rises above average, it is expected that diabetes is setting in. Early discovery reduces the chances of causing complications to the crucial organs like kidneys, nerves, eyes, and blood vessels.

There are several laboratory tests for diabetes, but they should give some signs before the test can be carried out. Our bodies function in various ways, and it provides mild to unnoticed symptoms of diabetes. Three types, which are type 1, type 2, and gestational diabetes. Type 2 diabetes may not be noticed on time, although Type 1 may give quick symptoms such as increased appetite, increased thirst, or polyphagia.

5.0.1 Testing Diabetes and Prediabetes Diagnosis

Fasting plasma glucose test

It detects prediabetes or diabetes. A fasting plasma glucose test is carried out at least on patients that haven't eaten for 8 hours. And afterwards, the blood glucose is measured.

The test is best carried out in the morning after a fasting period through the night. The values have different meanings, and they are used to classify the type of diabetes or prediabetes.

A fasting glucose level of 100 - 125mg/dL is at impaired fasting glucose (IFG). And this a prediabetes stage, meaning that patients with this value are more likely to develop type 2 diabetes although they do not have it yet. When the value rises above 126mg/dL, it means the patient has diabetes. And this must be confirmed with a repeated test in the following:

- Normal: 99 mg/dL and below
- Prediabetes: 100 - 125 mg/dL
- Diabetes: 126 and above

Random plasma glucose test

A random plasma glucose test is carried out on the patient without considering the last time he/she eats. It measures diabetes but cannot be used to test prediabetes. Additionally, it is not as reliable as a fasting glucose test. Although, the accuracy is reinforced by the assessment of symptoms after the random plasma glucose test. Symptoms are increased urination, increased thirst, and unexplained weight loss, fatigue, blurred vision, increased hunger, and sores that do not heal on time.

After the random plasma glucose test, other tests like FPG and OGTT are carried out to confirm the results of the random plasma glucose test, mostly the following day.

- Normal: N/A
- Prediabetes: N/A
- Diabetes: 200 mg/dl or above

Oral glucose tolerance test

The only difference between a fasting plasma glucose test, an oral glucose tolerance test is 2 hours of fasting after drinking the glucose-containing beverage. The patient undergoes 8 hours of fasting (like fasting plasma glucose test), followed by 2 hours of fasting again after drinking a glucose-containing beverage. This test is suitable to indicate diabetes or prediabetes.

Although OGTT is more challenging to administer, it is more sensitive and reliable than the FPG test for diagnosing prediabetes. OGTT is carried out after the patient has fasted for 8 hours, and the plasma glucose is measured. Then, the plasma glucose is measured again after two hours of fasting (when the patient must have taken glucose-containing drinks).

OGTT can be used to access gestational diabetes. In order to confirm this, blood sugar checks and analysis are carried out four times during the test, and if the patient blood is above normal at least twice during the test, the patient has gestational diabetes.

OGTT test for Gestational Diabetes:

- Fasting: 95 mg/dL or higher
- At 1 hour: 180 mg/dL or higher
- At 2 hours: 155 mg/dL or higher
- At 3 hours: 140 mg/dL or higher

A1C Test

The A1C test is a confirmation test and can be done without fasting. It works on the principle that a certain percentage of glucose is always attached to the hemoglobin. Since the average lifespan of the blood (where hemoglobin is located) is 120 days; then, A1C can measure the blood glucose level as far as 3 months back. A1C is used to monitor the status of blood glucose in diabetic patients so that the significance of the drugs prescribed can be observed and changed if it is mandatory.

- Normal: A1C below 5.7%
- Prediabetes: 5.7% - 6.4%
- Diabetes: 6.5% or above

5.0.2 Testing for Gestational Diabetes and Diagnosis

Gestation diabetes is diagnosed using blood samples. It is carried out between 24 and 28 weeks of pregnancy. Due to certain conditions such as the risk of getting a higher diabetes condition, the test may be carried out before the stated weeks. If the blood sugar is elevated at an early stage of pregnancy, it might be type 1 or type 2 pregnancy, unlike gestational diabetes, which is mostly at 24 - 28 weeks of pregnancy.

Glucose screening test

A glucose screening test is carried to measure the patient blood sugar. The patient takes a glucose drink, and after an hour, the blood sample is taken to check the blood level.

- Normal: 140 mg/dL or lower
- Higher: above 140 mg/dL

If the glucose level is increased or high, the patient will take a glucose tolerance test to confirm the diabetes condition.

Glucose tolerance test

It measures the blood sugar before and after taking a glucose drink. The patient fasts overnight and the blood sample is taken for the test. After the test, the patient drinks glucose-containing beverage and tests after 1 hour, 2 hours, and 3 hours afterward. The results can differ, and it is mandatory to check the standard measures of your institution.

5.1 Blood Test for Thyroid Function

Test for thyroid function is a way to know thyroid-stimulating hormone and thyroxine in the blood. An underactive thyroid means a change in the expected thyroid level in the blood; this can either be a high or low thyroid function level. A low level of thyroid-producing hormones, like triiodothyronine (T3) and thyroxine (T4), can change how the body processes fat. And this is why underactive thyroid (hypothyroidism) must be diagnosed at an early stage. Hypothyroidism can cause high cholesterol, atherosclerosis and this can cause the heart-related condition.

Both thyroid-stimulating hormone and T4 should be in a good and balanced state. If a patient shows high TSH with normal T4, the patient might develop underactive thyroid in the future. The patient should undergo a repeated blood test to finalize the check if he/she does not have an underactive thyroid.

Blood tests are likewise used to check some other thyroid tests, like knowing the level of triiodothyronine (T3) in the blood. Finally, a thyroid antibody test may be required after the usual thyroid test. This is applicable if the patient shows a high GP that suspects an autoimmune thyroid condition.

TSH tests

Changes in TSH occurs before the actual change in the level of thyroid hormone. So, TSH tests are first carried out to assess the thyroid hormone condition. This test is performed using patient blood samples.

Primary hypothyroidism is due to the point when the thyroid gland is not producing sufficient thyroid hormone, and a high TSH level indicates this condition. Also, low TSH shows that the body is producing too much thyroid hormone (hyperthyroidism). A high or low level of TSH might be a result of an abnormality in the pituitary gland. Any deviation from the typical values of 0.5 - 6 mill U/L is an abnormality in the thyroid hormone.

T4 tests

T4 is the thyroid hormone that flows in the blood.

Free T4 is the thyroid hormone that does not bound with any proteins and enters the body tissues quickly.

Bound T4 is the thyroid hormone bound to proteins and does not move freely in the body tissues.

Total T4 is the combination of free T4 and bound T4. These measures change when the bidding protein differs.

Primary hypothyroidism occurs when the level of TSH is high with low FT4 or FTI. And this can be due to disease in the thyroid gland. Also, hyperthyroidism is due to low TSH and high FT4 or FTI. This condition is due to hepatitis acute, thyroiditis, and hyperthyroidism

Hypothyroidism is due to low TSH and low FT4 or FTI. This condition is caused by chronic thyroiditis, cretinism, hypothyroidism, cirrhosis, and malnutrition.

- The normal range is 4 - 12 ug/dl

T3 tests

Mostly, T3 tests are used to diagnose the severity of hyperthyroidism. The patient with hyperthyroidism condition has a high T3 level. Some patients may have average FT4 or FTI, low TSH, with high T3.

A patient with hypothyroidism can have low FT4 or FTI, high TSH, with normal T3.

5.1.1 Non-Blood Test for Thyroid Function

Radioactive Iodine Uptake

The thyroid follows a particular mechanism through which it absorbs iodine from the bloodstream. The thyroid needs iodine to be able to carry out its regular activities, and T4 (thyroid hormone in the blood) contains iodine. So, the thyroid gland must take a certain amount of iodine in the bloodstream in other to produce T4.

Radioactive iodine can be used to measure the amount of iodine absorbed by the thyroid gland, and in turn, know the absorption rate and where it is explicitly absorbed. High RAIU is noticed in patients with overactive thyroid gland – hyperthyroidism. And low RAIU is seen in patients with underactive thyroid gland – hypothyroidism.

A thyroid scan can be used to display the level and mode of intake/absorption. This will show a picture of the thyroid gland and reveals what parts of the thyroid absorbed the iodine.

5.2 Test for Parathyroid Functions

Behind the thyroid gland there are four-sectioned parathyroid glands located. This hormone regulates calcium, phosphorus levels, and vitamin D in the blood and bones. The regulation of calcium levels in the blood through the parathyroid hormone is used to monitor or test for parathyroid functions. The secretion of PTH is affected by the level of calcium in the blood. A high level of calcium promotes slow secretion of PTH, and a low level causes the parathyroid gland to produce more PTH. When the calcium blood level is not balanced, it can be a result of a clinical issue with the parathyroid gland or PTH.

Heavy calcium in the blood can be an indicator of hyperparathyroidism – this is seen when the parathyroid is overactive and it produces too much PTH. This can cause irregular heartbeats, brain abnormalities, and kidney stones.

A low or reduced level of calcium in the blood can be a sign of hypoparathyroidism – a condition of underactive parathyroid glands that cannot produce enough PTH.

Osteomalacia, muscle spasms, heart rhythm disturbances, and tetany are considered to be signs of hypoparathyroidism.

Some of these applications are used to determine the parathyroid test function. Which are:

- Determination of non-responding osteoporosis treatment
- Determination of cause of low phosphorus levels in the blood
- Monitoring effectiveness of treatment in parathyroid-related issues
- Check parathyroid function
- Know the differences between parathyroid and non-parathyroid-related disorders

Procedure for a PTH test

The test is similar to a blood test, and it might require excellent venipuncture skills. The blood is tested for various levels of elements that indicate a low/high PTH amount, as mentioned above.

A low level of PTH can indicate:

- Autoimmune disorder
- Radiation exposure to the parathyroid glands
- Vitamin D intoxication
- Hypoparathyroidism
- Spread of cancer to the bone
- Sarcoidosis
- Low serum magnesium

A high level of PTH can indicate:

- Hyperparathyroidism (however, if the PTH level is normal and the calcium levels are low, it might not be due to apathy glands malfunction but due to other causes)
- Tumors in parathyroid glands
- Pregnancy, which is quite uncommon
- Chronic kidney disease
- Lack of calcium (either the patient is not taking enough calcium, or the body is not absorbing calcium, or such loses calcium through urine)
- Vitamin D disorder

5.3 Tests for adrenal function

Adrenal function tests may be hard to diagnose at the early stage of adrenal insufficiency. Patient medical history (including present signs and symptoms) may give an insight on adrenal function or otherwise. Notable test to verify adrenal function includes; a blood test. ACTH stimulation test, insulin-induced hypoglycemia test, and imaging tests.

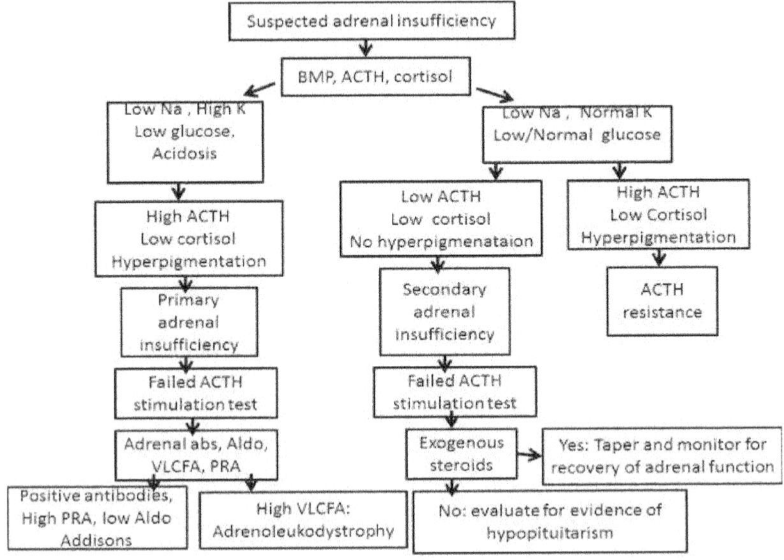

ACTH stimulation test

From a diagnosis standpoint, this test helps to check the adrenal gland's response to exogenous ACTH. The mode and degree of test/response are measured by physiologic integrity of the gland and also the stimulation.

Based on measuring the cortisol level, the ACTH test is used to diagnose adrenal function by accessing the androgen precursor levels.

For the fast ACTH test, a couple of blood tests are gathered to decide basal degrees of plasma cortisol, trailed by intravenous infusion of 250 μg cosyntropin. Plasma might be examined 30 minutes, 45 minutes, or an hour after ACTH administration. With a typical reaction to incitement, the plasma cortisol level will surpass 15 μg/dl and will display a gradual ascent of 5–7 μg/dl or more. A typical response prohibits essential adrenocortical deficiency. Notwithstanding, it does not bar halfway optional adrenocortical inadequacy; patients with mild or early ACTH insufficiency may have adequate basal ACTH creation to forestall adrenocortical loss.

Delayed ACTH incitement may likewise recognize essential from auxiliary adrenocortical deficiency. One convention for delayed ACTH incitement is an assortment of 24-hour urine examples for 1 day before ACTH incitement and the 2 days during ACTH implantation to decide the estimations of 17-OHCS and creatinine.107 A nonstop intravenous mixture of 1600 μg cosyntropin, comparable to the 160 units of ACTH initially utilized, is directed 48 hours. It is not vital to limit diet or action during the mixture.

Typical subjects discharge over 27 mg/24 hours 17-OHCS on the primary day of the implantation and above 47 mg/24 hours on a subsequent day. Patients with auxiliary adrenocortical deficiency by and large discharge above 4 mg/24 hours on the principal day of implantation and above 10 mg/24 hours on a subsequent day. Patients with essential adrenocortical deficiency, as a rule, discharge under 3 mg/24 hours right off the bat and under 4 mg/24 hours on the second.

In patients with essential adrenal deficiency, glucocorticoid treatment might be started at the hour of a fast ACTH incitement test or during a drawn-out ACTH incitement convention. Dexamethasone is the glucocorticoid of decision; it is multiple times stronger than cortisol, and the sum needed for treatment does not meddle with cortisol or 17-OHCS assurance. Although dexamethasone stifles the pituitary emission of endogenous ACTH, it doesn't interfere with the adrenal reaction to exogenous ACTH and subsequently won't change the test's consequences.

The ACTH incitement tests for the finding of CAH include the estimation of steroid antecedents proximal to the enzymatic square. Different conventions have been utilized. Some requirements for the time being dexamethasone concealment before testing, albeit most clinicians don't think about this progression as significant.

Levels of progesterone and 17-OH progesterone are raised with CAH21, the degree of coursing 18-deoxycorticosterone is presented with CAH11, and the 17-hydroxypregnenolone:17-hydroxyprogesterone proportion is raised with CAH3β-HSD.

Insulin tolerance test

Insulin tolerance test is applicable if the first ACTH approach is not satisfactory or if the results show some significant problems linked to the pituitary.

The test is carried out by administering an IV injection of insulin (this injection lowers blood sugar level). Hypoglycemia is vulnerable to set in. Therefore, the administration needs to be monitored. Once the injection is administered, it causes stress, which induces the secretion of ACTH from the pituitary gland. The patient blood should be taken and tested, followed by other blood extractions every 30 minutes for the next 2 hours after the first test. Insulin tolerance test is the reliable way to check and confirm secondary adrenal insufficiency. If the cortisol is low, it means the adrenal is producing enough cortisol because the pituitary is not making enough ACTH.

ITT should not be performed on patients with heart disease, seizures, and some other chronic diseases. ITT makes the blood sugar drop to the low range, and it is dangerous for patients with such a condition. Proper monitoring should be done on the patient through the test period.

CRH stimulation test

This test is considered to be another option to carry out secondary insufficiency test of the adrenal function of ACTH test do not give a precise result. The CRH stimulation test is a confirmation test to differentiate secondary adrenal function to tertiary adrenal function.

The patient is injected with an IV injection of CRH, and the sample is tested in a period of 30 minutes, 60 minutes, 90 minutes, and 120 minutes after the injection to measure ACTH level.

Non-responsive ACTH production after CRH injection shows secondary adrenal function. And the slow response of ACTH production to CRH injection shows tertiary adrenal insufficiency.

https://www.semanticscholar.org/paper/5fe597829d6859a84190cf47e71310426588b72c

Chapter 6: Renal Function tests

The kidney is a crucial organ that plays a role in removing renal waste products like urea, creatinine, and uric acid. Moreover, it plays a role in balancing extracellular fluid, serum osmolality, and electrolyte concentrations. The renal function test is significant in managing patients with kidney disease or any renal related functions. The test has the option to cover up the renal disease, monitoring the kidney response in patients, and determination of renal disease in a patient.

Specimen collection

Specimen collection from patient varies according to the type of renal test that has to be carried out. A blood sample is sufficient or adequate enough to carry out serum creatinine and blood urea nitrogen (BUN) on a patient. Notwithstanding, the outcomes may not be accurate if the patient eat proteins close to the test period. This is because proteins increase serum creatinine and urea levels to a significant level in the blood. And also, BUN measurements may be affected by hydration status. The patient must be kept at a suitable hydration level so that accurate results can be obtained.

Time is a significant measure in urine samples, valued in 24-hour time, like urine creatinine clearance. The sample must be taken at the right time – over or under collection may affect the final results. A minimum of 5 hours and a maximum of 8 hours is preferable to a 24-hour collection.

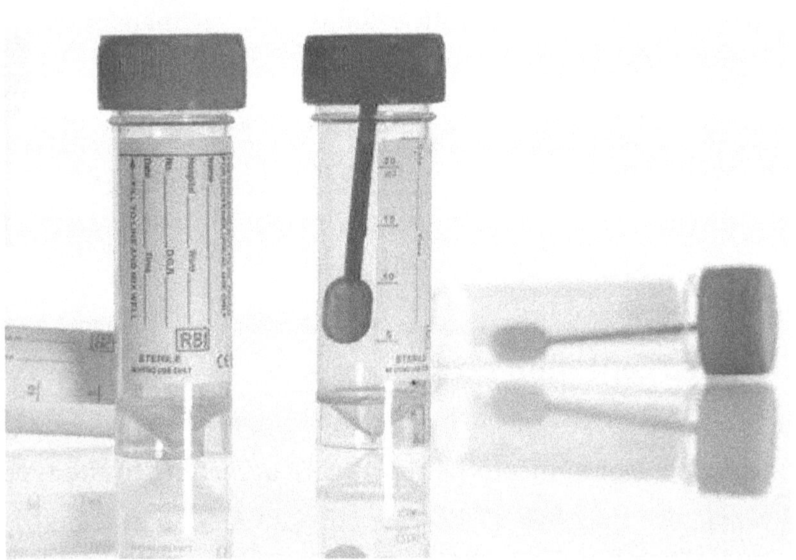

Procedures

Many approaches are suitable to access clinical laboratory tests for renal function. They are all significantly crucial by determining the level of glomerular filtration rate (GFR) and check for proteinuria (albuminuria).

- *Urine test.* ACR is "albumin-to-creatinine ratio." Albumin is a protein found mainly in the blood, as the body needs it. It is founded in the blood but not in the urine since the kidney filters it off. When this protein (albumin) is found in the urine, it means the kidney is not performing its function hundred percent. That's why the urine test for ACR is a way to check and confirm kidney disease. The renal function test is carried out for over three months, and if it is positive, that is a confirmation of kidney disease.

- *Blood test.* Creatinine is a waste that comes from the muscle into the blood. Kidney filters off this waste and makes the blood free of it. If damaged, the kidney will have problems eliminating this waste, and a creatinine test is the first step to take in testing for glomerular filtration rate. After all the tests, the gathered results are used to calculate the GFR, and this shows how well the kidney is working.

Glomerular Filtration Rate

The best in the general pointer of the glomerular capacity is the glomerular filtration rate (GFR). GFR is the rate in milliliters every moment at which substances in plasma are separated through the glomerulus; at the end of the day, the clear image of a substance from the blood.

The typical GFR for a grown-up male is 90 to 120 mL for every moment. The attributes of a perfect or ideal marker of GFR are as per the following:

- It shows up in the plasma at a consistent rate
- It openly filtered at the glomerulus
- The renal tube does not absorb or discharge GFR
- GFR does not go through extra-renal disposal.

As no such endogenous marker right now exists, exogenous markers of GFR are utilized. Appraisal of GFR utilizing inulin, a polysaccharide, is viewed as the reference technique for the assessment of GFR. It includes the implantation of inulin and afterward the estimation of blood levels after a predefined period to decide the pace of inulin leeway. Other used exogenous markers are radioisotopes, for example, chromium-51 ethylene-diamine-tetra-acidic corrosive (51 Cr-EDTA), and technetium-99-named diethylene-triamine-pentaacetate (99 Tc-DTPA). The most encouraging exogenous marker is the non-radioactive differentiation specialist, iohexol, particularly in kids.

The bother related with the utilization of exogenous markers, explicitly that the testing must be acted in particular places, and the trouble to examine these substances, has energized the utilization of endogenous markers.

Creatinine

The most ordinarily utilized endogenous marker for the evaluation of glomerular capacity is creatinine. The determined leeway of creatinine is utilized to give a marker of GFR. This includes the assortment of urine over a 24-hour term or ideally over a precisely planned time of 5 to 8 hours, since 24-hour assortments are famously inconsistent.

Creatinine clearance is then determined utilizing the formula:

C = (U x V)/P

C = freedom, U = urinary focus, V = urinary stream rate (volume/time for example ml/min), and P = plasma fixation

Creatinine clearance ought to be rectified for body surface territory. Ill-advised or deficient urine assortment is one of the significant issues influencing this test's accuracy; subsequently, the planned assortment is valuable. Besides, because of rounded discharge, creatinine overestimates GFR by around 10% to 20%.

Blood Urea Nitrogen (BUN)

BUN is a waste product that is accumulated in the liver and excreted by the kidney. It is a waste of protein metabolism and urea cycle—meaning it cannot be overruled unless it is taken care of. Although the kidney does not excrete all the area, it contributes to over 85% of the excretion, and the gastrointestinal tract removes the rest. The level of urea serum rises in a patient when the kidney fails to excrete the large percentage. Although other conditions like GI bleeding, dehydration, high protein digestion, and catabolic states can increase the urea level in the blood. Likewise, urea can be decreased in starvation, low protein consumption, and severe liver disease.

Blood urea nitrogen is not as accurate as the test for serum creatinine. Still, it is a significant symptom of early renal disease (as blood urea increases in renal disease).

- **Bun ratio: creatine**

  The BUN ratio can be useful to differentiate pre-renal from the renal causes when blood urea increased. In pre-renal disease conditions, the level of BUN ratio is 20:1. And the intrinsic renal disease is closer to 10:1.

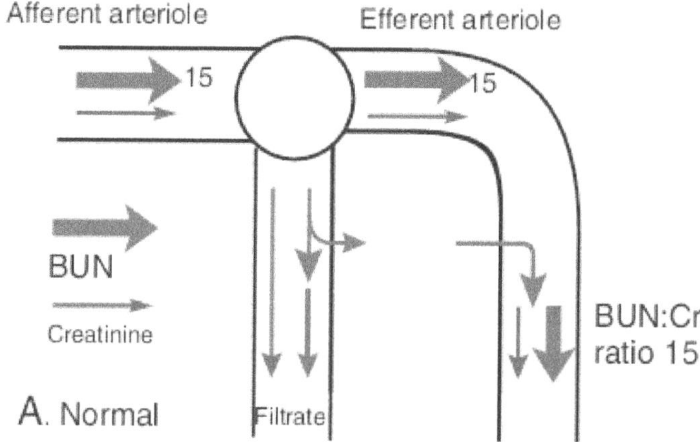

Cystatin C

Cystatin C is a protein that functions as a protease inhibitor produced by all the body nucleated cells. It is a low-molecular-weight protein and formed at different rates in the body and the kidney filters it. Cystatin C's level is an inverse of GFR – high-level Cystatin C shows low GFR and vice versa. Unlike GFR, when the kidney (glomeruli) filter Cystatin C off the body, it is reabsorbed by the proximal renal tubules. Regularly, Cystatin C does not enter the urine, as it is filtered off. The amount of Cystatin C can be measured in the blood and the urine.

https://doi.org/10.7326%2F0003-4819-158-11-201306040-00007

https://web.archive.org/web/20160324124828/http://humanphysiology.tuars.com/program/section7/7ch04/7ch04p11.htm

http://content.nejm.org/cgi/pmidlookup?view=short&pmid=8366899&promo=ONFLNS19

Chapter 7: Liver tests and Gastrointestinal Function tests

Liver tests are grouped into many test functions, and each of them has various essential parameters in order to detect the information about the liver. Some of the tests are prothrombin time, albumin, bilirubin, and many more. The liver transaminases aspartate (AST) are beneficial biomarkers in the liver that are used to detect liver injury in patients that show symptoms of liver dysfunction. Liver diseases do not always show significant signs, most of the times are mild ones, and they must be seen early enough for better results and treatments. Liver test functions are carried out in the blood (then the patient blood is taken as a sample in the laboratory), albumin (the test for liver functionality through the albumin), transaminase (the test for the cellular integrity of the liver through the use of transaminase), and gamma-glutamyl transferase and alkaline phosphatase (the test on the biliary tract of the liver).

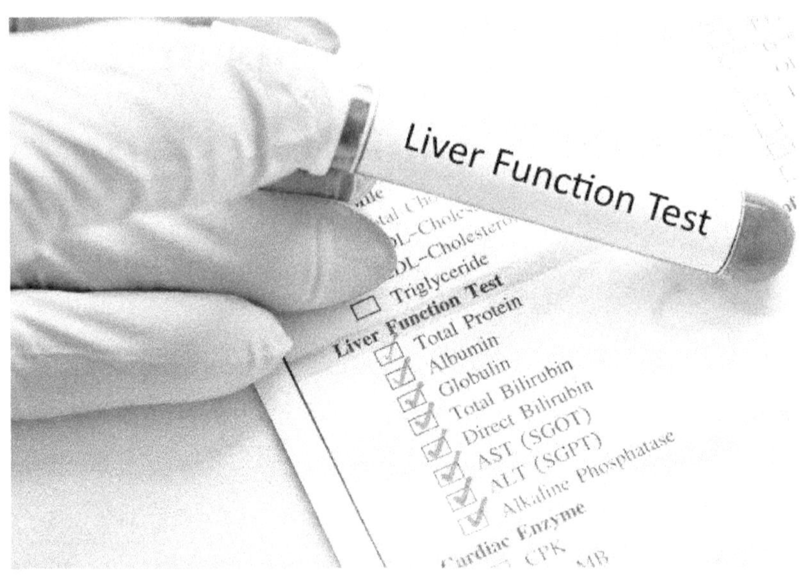

Clinically, these tests are more linked to liver chemistries rather than to liver functions, as most of these tests do not measure the "functionality of the liver." More than just one test is carried out on a patient with hepatic dysfunction to measure and evaluate biochemical tests in the patient. The test shows differences in liver disease and distinguish all type of liver disorders, give insight on the extent of liver damage, and overall progression in the treatment of the liver disease. The test is usually carried out twice a year, and this is purposely used to monitor the progress of the patient in response to treatments, mostly on those that are taking certain medications, such as anticonvulsants.

7.1 Liver Test

Total bilirubin

Measuring the level of bilirubin is in two stages: the measurement of conjugated and unconjugated bilirubin. The unconjugated bilirubin forms substances from the breakdown product of heme – a part in the red blood cell, specifically hemoglobin. The unconjugated bilirubin is not soluble because it is not water-soluble. The function of the liver is to make it soluble and convert it to conjugated bilirubin through an enzyme – UDP-glucuronyl-transferase.

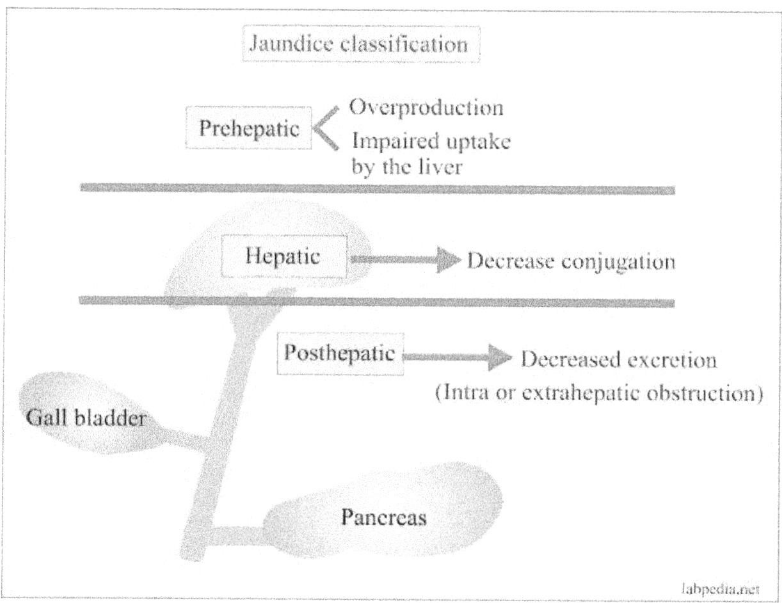

Liver disease is confirmed in patients with a total bilirubin that is above 17 umol/L. Jaundice is confirmed when the total bilirubin level is above 40umol/L.

If the unconjugated bilirubin increases, it is due to less overproduction of unconjugated bilirubin, less conversion to conjugated form, and reduced absorption of conjugated bilirubin by the liver. Clinically, the overproduction of bilirubin is due to the reabsorption of hematoma, leading to ineffective erythropoiesis, which later increases the destruction of the red blood cells.

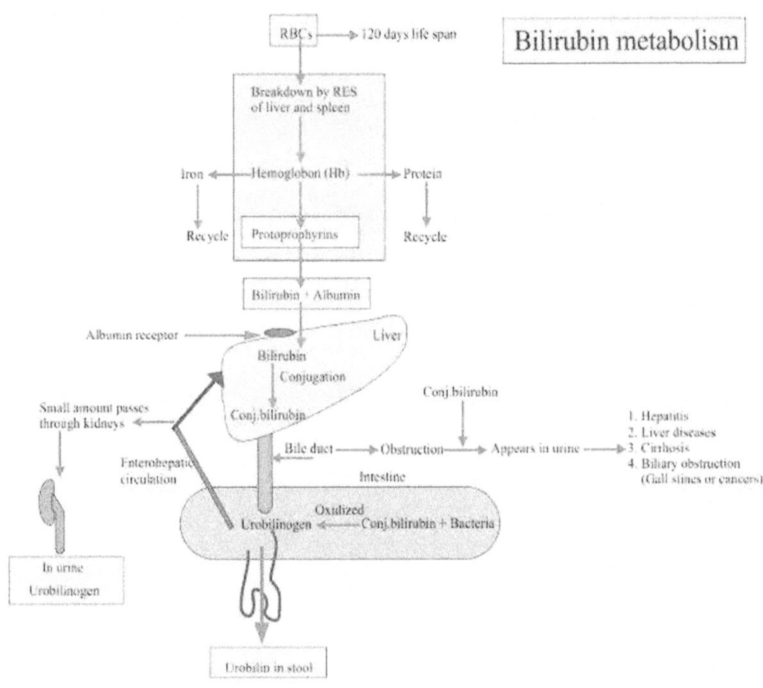

The amount of rising in conjugated bilirubin is directly proportional to the level of hepatocyte injury. Moreover, viral hepatitis can increase the conjugated bilirubin level.

The measurements of bilirubin level vary in newborn babies. Bilimeter is used in testing for bilirubin on newborns instead of the LFTs. Also, a transcutaneous bilirubin meter can be used instead of a bilimeter. Hyperbilirubinemia occurs in newborns when its level rises above the 95th percentile during the first week of life. Light therapy is applicable in newborns to reduce the amount of bilirubin in the blood. When the blood bilirubin rises above 5 mg/dL per day, and conjugated bilirubin is dark, then serum bilirubin is more than normal physiological range, and pathological jaundice should be suspected in newborns.

Albumin

The liver explicitly produces albumin, and its measurements are not hard and cheaply done. The total component of albumin is a protein (although with minor constituents of globulins).

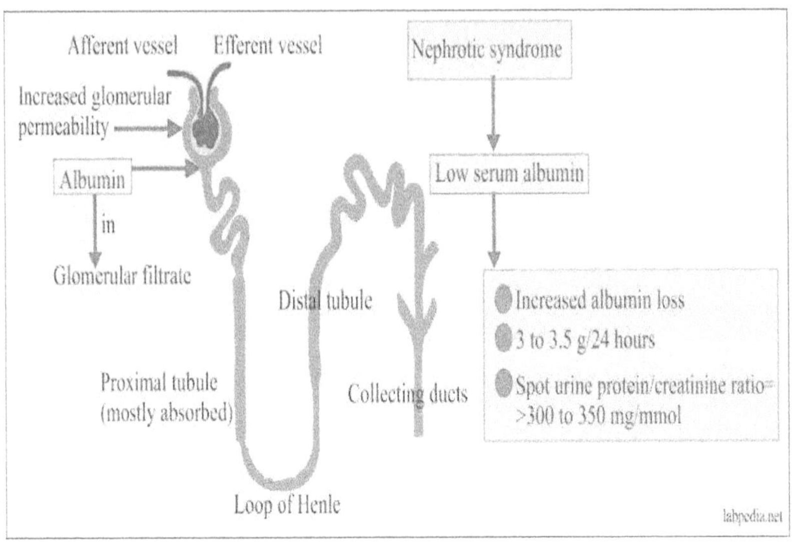

Reduced albumin is noticed in patients with chronic liver disease like hepatitis, cirrhosis, and ascites; in kidney diseases like glomerulonephritis and nephropathy; malnutrition, malabsorption syndromes, burn injuries, and nephrotic syndrome where it is lost through the blood. In low albumin, the intravascular oncotic pressure is lower than the extravascular space; thus, low albumin contributes to *edema*.

A high level of albumin is also noticed in dehydration.

Alkaline phosphatase (ALP)

Alkaline phosphatase is found in various parts of the linings in the organs. It is an enzyme found in the cells lining the biliary ducts of the liver and the lining of the small intestine, liver, placenta, and kidneys. The bone aids about half the percentage of the blood ALP activities. It plays a role in the calcification of the bones and transposition of the small intestines.

Causes of high increase in ALP are: infiltrative liver diseases, granulomatous liver disease, amyloidosis, and abscess. Low ALP levels are seen in a patient with zinc deficiency, hypophosphatasia, hypothyroidism, and pernicious anemia.

In pregnancy, ALP increases in the third trimester. Hyperemesis gravidarum causes ALP to grow to over 215 IU/L, meanwhile in pre-eclampsia ALP, about 14 IU/L, and as for HELLP syndrome, ALP levels can get up to 15 IU/L.

Aspartate transaminase (AST)

AST has two isoenzymes, which are found in the mitochondria and cytoplasmic. AST is located in the kidney, brain, pancreas, lungs, heart, muscle, and liver in high concentration. The wide range of the isoenzymes makes it a less specific indicators of liver damage. More percentage of liver AST is given by mitochondria AST forms of the isoenzymes. The cytoplasmic form contributes to the circulating AST blood.

Decreased values of AST may be observed in congested liver or patients with high cholesterol levels.
Increased values are due to liver disease, high alcohol consumption, kidney infections, myocardial infarction.

Test with AST should be confirmed together with other tests, as high or low AST can indicate other organs' diseases.

Alanine transaminase (ALT)

Alanine transaminase catalyzes the transamination reaction and is found only in the cytoplasmic form. ALT is found in the kidney, heart, and muscles, although it is found in high concentration in the liver.

When ALT is above 300 IU/L, it is not specificly due to the liver and can pose a threat to other organs in the body.

When ALT is above 500 IU/L, the causes are usually due to the liver and can be caused by hepatitis, ischemic liver injury, and high toxins in the liver. Hepatitis A, B, C are different, and they rise differently in the blood. ALT levels in Hepatitis C rise more than in Hepatitis A and B. Other things that contribute to high ALT are: alcohol liver disease & non-alcoholic fatty liver disease; fat accumulation in the liver during childhood obesity, abs steatohepatitis. Triglycerides, reduced glucose tolerance, decreased insulin response and increased free fatty acids are associated with rising ALT.

ALT rises during the second trimester in pregnancy and reduces by about 50% after child delivery.

ALT/AST ratio

The ALT/AST ratio increases in liver functional impairment. The ratio is more significant than 1.17 in viral cirrhosis, 1.45 in alcoholic liver disease, ratio 1.33 in post necrotic liver cirrhosis, more significant than 2.0 in alcoholic hepatitis, and 0.9 in non-alcoholic hepatitis.

Gamma-glutamyl transpeptidase (GGT)

GGT aids in glutathione metabolism, where it transports peptides across the cell membrane. GGT is mostly found in hepatocytes, renal tubules, pancreas, biliary epithelial cells, and intestines.

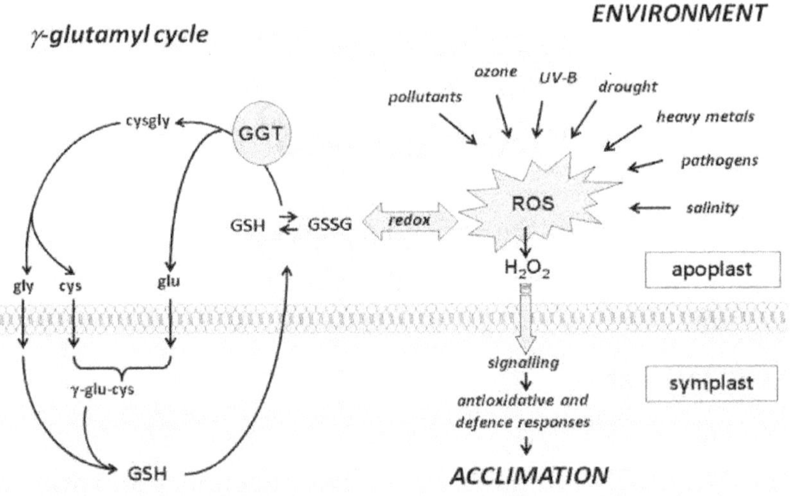

Like ALP, GGT increases in viral hepatitis, especially with hepatitis C. It rises about 10 times in alcoholic consumption. About 50% increase in patients with the non-alcoholic liver disease.

Other causes of high GGT are myocardial infarction, hyperthyroidism, obesity, diabetes mellitus, acute pancreatitis, myotonic dystrophy, and Guillain-Barré syndrome.

Ceruloplasmin

Ceruloplasmin is an acute-phase protein synthesized in the liver. It carries copper ions and increases in infection, pregnancy, rheumatoid arthritis, and obstructive jaundice.

Coagulation test

The liver produces the majority of coagulation factors. An international normalized ratio (INR) is used to monitor coagulation problems in patients. Elevated INR is noticed in a patient with liver disease, but this does not show that the patient is potentially bleeding; this test only measures the procoagulants and not anticoagulants. Despite an elevated INR in liver disease, the synthesis of procoagulants and anticoagulants both decreases, some patient even shows hypercoagulable.

Alpha-fetoprotein

AFP is seen in the fetal liver. The mechanism and biochemical process that leads to a decrease in AFP is not known in adults. Mostly, the liver's exposure to cancer-causing agents and seize liver maturation in childhood can lead to increased AFP.

https://www.letsgetchecked.com/articles/how-often-should-you-get-liver-function-check/

Chapter 8: Test for Malignancies

Various tests are carried out on patients to test for the presence of cancer using laboratory measures. Most of the tests are conducted via samples of blood, urine, and other significant body fluids, which are used to determine if a patient has the disease or pre-cancerous conditions. These tests are also used to check if the patient is responding to treatments, to check the level of cancerous therapy, the stage of the cancer, and to identify the right treatment options. Laboratory tests are also used to check if a patient has a cancer recurrence – this is a condition where a new cancer or disease returned to its original location.

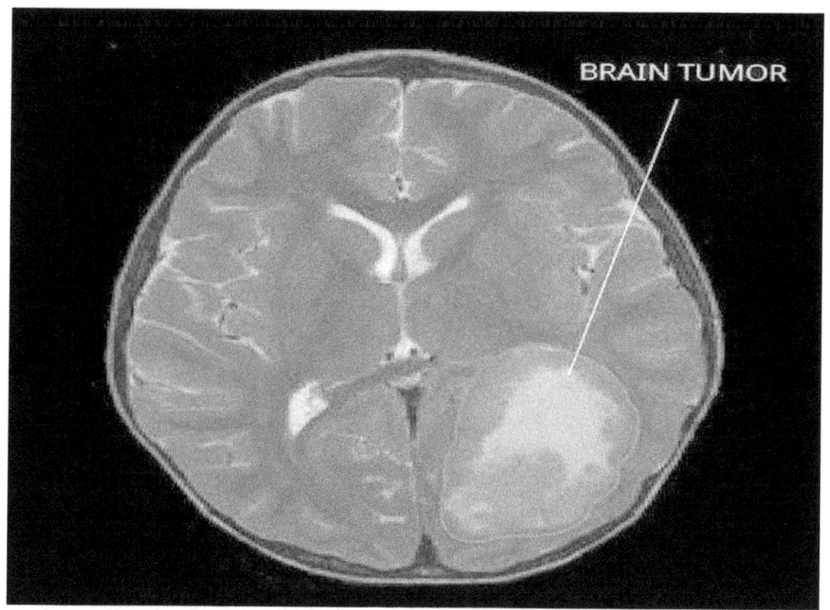

8.1 Tumor markers

Tumor markers are produced in the body (in high quantity) when cancer or cancerous substances are present in the body. Mostly, they are found in the blood, tumor tissues, stool, and urine. Tumor markers are often proteins, but DNA changes might occur, or the gene changes in green expression pattern due to the cancerous factors.

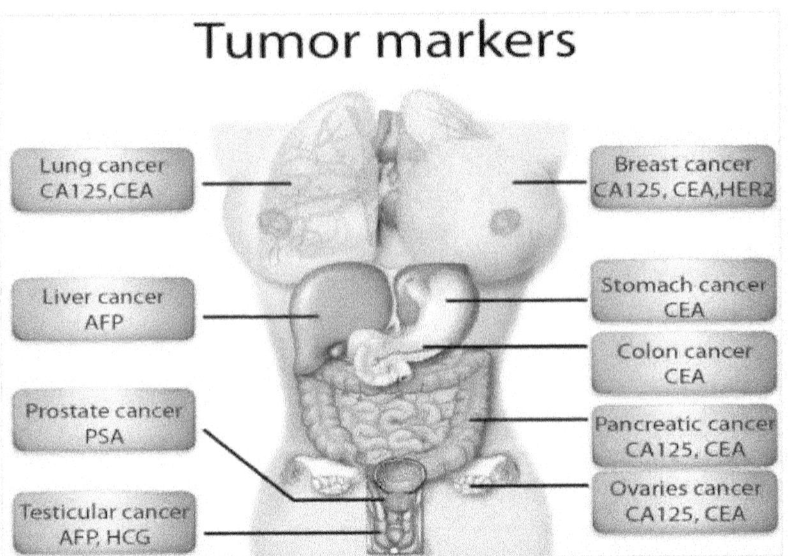

Clinically, tumor markers alone cannot measure or give a concise value about cancer or a pre-cancerous condition. Therefore, they are used alongside other measurements to provide good readings to testing tumors.

The role of tumor markers includes:

- Screening of patient for malignances
- To evaluate the stage of the tumor and assessing prognosis.
- Diagnosing specific tumor types in case biopsy is not feasible.
- Monitoring patient that has undergone a cancer treatment

CA-125 Test

CA-125 is a protein tumor marker, that is found in higher concentration in cancer cells – majorly ovarian cancer cells. The CA-125 test is used to measure the number of cancer antigens in a patient's blood.

CA-125 is higher than the normal range when some cancer types occure, such as: ovarian, colon, breast, lung, stomach, pancreatic, fallopian tube, endometrial, liver, lung, and esophageal. Also, cancer that grows to the peritoneum and abdominal lining may increase the level of CA-125 in a patient.

Other conditions that can increase CA-125, aside from a tumor or cancerous cells, are endometriosis, lupus, pancreatitis, liver disease, and uterine fibroids.

Prostate-specific antigen test

The prostate gland produces PSA. The prostate antigen test measures the level of PSA in the blood. A high PSA level may be an indication of prostate cancer. It can also indicate a non-cancerous condition like benign prostatic hyperplasia and prostatitis.

Patients with a high level of PSA or PSA symptoms are treated with a digital rectal exam (DRE).

National Cancer Institute research shows that patients with a low PSA level have prostate cancer, and high PSA patients do not have it.

Marker	Cancer type	Tests	Notes
Beta-2-microglobulin	Chronic lymphocytic, multiple myeloma, and some lymphomas	Spinal fluid, blood, and urine	The test is used to check treatment progression and prognosis
CA15-3/CA27.29	Breast cancer	Blood	The test is used to check treatment progression and diagnose cancer recurrence

Alpha-fetoprotein	Liver cancer	Blood	The test is used to check treatment progression, used to know the diagnose and stage of cancer, and determine the choice of treatment
Beta-human chorionic gonadotropin	Choriocarcinoma and germ cell tumors	Blood or Urine	The test is used to check treatment progression, used to know the diagnose and stage of cancer, and determine the choice of treatment

HE4	Ovarian cancer	Blood	The test is used to check treatment progression, used to know the diagnose cancer reoccurrence, and determine the choice of treatment
Carcinoembryonic antigen	Colorectal cancer	Blood	The test is used to check treatment progression, used to know the diagnose and stage of cancer, and determine the choice of treatment

Chromogranin A	Neuroendocrine tumors	Blood	Tests may be used to determine treatment options, monitor for recurrence band measure the response to treatment.
Calcitonin	Thyroid cancer	Blood	Tests may be used to determine treatment options, monitor for recurrence band measure the response to treatment.

Immunoglobulins	Multiple myeloma and non-Hodgkin lymphoma	Urine and Blood	Tests may be used to determine treatment options, monitor for recurrence band measure the response to treatment.
Thyroglobulin	Thyroid cancer	Blood	Tests may be used to determine treatment options, monitor for recurrence band measure the response to treatment.

Neuron-specific enolase	Lung cancer	Blood	Tests may be used to determine treatment options, monitor for recurrence band measure the response to treatment.
CA 19-9	Bile duct cancer, gastric cancer, gallbladder, pancreatic cancer, and bile duct cancer	Blood	Tests may help measure the response to treatment
Nuclear matrix protein	Bladder cancer	Urine	The test may be used to measure treatment. Ki

CTC test

Circulating tumor cells detach from the located cells and enter the bloodstream. Circulating tumor cell (CTC) tests can trace or monitor metastatic breast, prostate, and colorectal cancers. This test allows us to capture, count, and identify circulating tumor cells in the blood sample. The blood test is carried out before the therapy or during the treatment.

Flow cytometry

Flow cytometry holds the properties of cells in sample of bone marrow, lymph hubs, or blood. The sample is first treated with unique antibodies and passed before a laser pillar. If the antibodies append to the cells, the cells radiate light. The presence of specific substances, or antigens, on the outside of cells, may help recognize the cell type.

Flow cytometry may likewise be utilized to gauge the measure of DNA in malignancy cells. For this situation, the cells are treated with great light-touchy colors that respond with DNA.

This test is utilized to analyze and arrange certain malignant growths, for example leukemia and lymphoma, and to assess the danger of reappearance. Flow cytometry likewise might be utilized as a component of the undifferentiated organism transplantation measure.

Complete blood count test

Complete blood count test is the measurements of the blood cells that are circulating the bloodstream. In particular, it gauges a blood test for the degree of red platelets, which convey oxygen all through the body; white platelets, which help with blood coagulating. The test additionally gauges hemoglobin, a protein in red platelets that conveys oxygen, and hematocrit, the proportion of red platelets to plasma.

A CBC might be utilized to distinguish an assortment of conditions, including leukemia, sickliness, and contamination. Likewise, because some malignant growth medicines may incidentally bring down blood tallies, oncologists regularly use CBC tests all through treatment to intently screen a patient's blood checks.

The Oncotype test

The Oncotype DX lab test is used to decide if chemotherapy is probably going to profit patients with beginning phase lower malignant growth. It likewise assesses the probability of infection repetition.

This demonstrative test is frequently performed on a modest quantity of tissue eliminated during lower disease medical procedure and afterward analyzed at a sub-atomic level.

The Oncotype DX test gives detailed data about the sickness, which may help control therapy choices.

Mammaprint + Blueprint test

The Mammaprint 70-Gene Breast Cancer Recurrence Assay might be utilized to decide the danger or possibility that a patient's disease will return. A high-hazard score implies the malignancy has a three-in-10 possibility of returning. A good outcome places the odds at one out of 10. Neither one of the results indicates that the threat will or will not return, yet the evaluation might be utilized to establish treatment choices.

The Blueprint 80-Gene Molecular Subtyping Assay inspects which of the tumor's transformations are directing the malignancy's conduct. When utilized with the Mammaprint measure, Blueprint may characterize every tumor into a subtype characterization, which may help manage treatment choices.

http://seer.cancer.gov/statfacts/html/all.html

Chapter 9: Urine and Stool Analysis

Urine analysis is always done before a surgery or medical test to confirm some symptoms or suspects of a disease. The test is useful as an essential tool in checking for elements for both renal and systemic pathologies. The urinalysis part can be done using urine dipsticks—and a change in colors reads the test.

Some of the components that contribute to the examination of urine and color changes are:

- Blood cells, as an indicator of internal bleeding or urinary tract infection, respectively.
- Alkalines, proteins, electrolytes, and acids used to monitor fluid balance and kidney function in a patient
- Infection diseases parameters and pathogens: this is used to find the source of an infection in a patient
- Tumor markers: for example, the presence of hormones like catecholamines in the urine is associated with a malignant disease—neuroblastoma.
- Glucose: to discover overdose in glucocorticoids during some specific treatment and to monitor kidney function in patients.

9.1 Gross Visual Analysis

Some physical and psychological feelings are used to distinguish urine.

Odor

Urinalysis is performed by observing the odor of the urine. Normal urine smells like "nutty"; the deviation may imply some illness.

Fruity smell shows the presence of ketone bodies in the urine. And it is observed in starving patients, dehydration, or uncontrolled diabetes.

The sweet smell is an indication of maple syrup urine disease.

The fetid odor is an indication of E.coli infection.

A mousy or musty odor is an indication of phenylketonuria.

Appearance and color

The color of urine varies, and the average color is yellow due to the presence of urochrome. The color can change with different ranges like pale, dark, or deep amber, or straw-colored – urine color changes due to the accumulation of drugs, water, foods, or special medical conditions.

Urine clarity is aided by the substances in the urine, and they include debris, casts, proteins, bacteria, and crystals. This clarity can be described as clear, cloudy, turbid, and mildly cloudy.

Urine color	Condition	Foods	Drugs
Black	Alkaptonuria Malignant melanoma	Non	Non
Red	Hemoglobinuria	Beets	Chlorpromazine

Blue	Tryptophan malabsorption	Non	Methylene blue Indomethacin Amitriptyline
Brown	Hepatobiliary disease Gilbert syndrome Tyrosinemia	Feva beans	Metronidazole Levodopa Nitrofurantoi n Chloroquine
Purple	Bacteria - seen in a patient with indwelling catheters	Non	Non
Orange	Non	Vitamins C, Carrots, and fatty foods	Phenazopyridi ne Rifampicin

Green	Urinary tract infection	Asparagus	Propofol Vitamin B
White	Chyluria Phosphatase crystals Pyuria	Non	Propofol

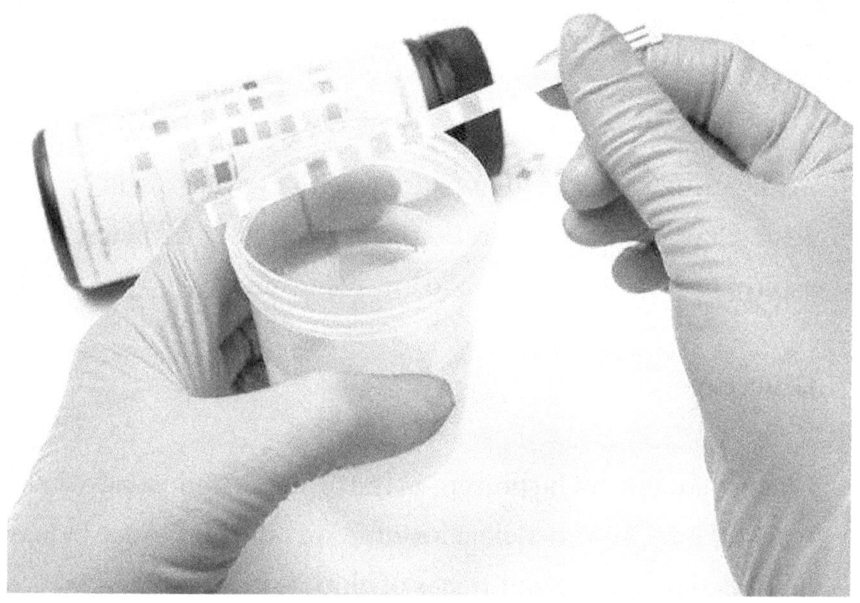

pH

pH varies in concentration and is analyzed as either basic, alkaline, or neutral. The normal pH of urine is 4.6 - 8.0.

Alkaline urine shows in patients with a high concentration of basic substances like calcium phosphate and magnesium ammonium phosphate. It is also observed if the patient's renal calculi are made of these substances. Alkaline urine can occur due to kidney infection, asthma, urinary tract infection, or severe vomiting.

Acidic urine is observed in patients with cystine calculi or uric acid. Starvation, dehydration, uncontrolled diabetes, and aspirin overdose contribute to low pH urine.

Glucose

Glucose should not be present in the urine, as it must have been reabsorbed. But, deficiencies due to infection or kidney malfunction may permit traces of glucose in it.

A high cluster of glucose in the blood, like above 180 mg/dl, permits the kidney to release some quantity into the urine, as excreting automatically. It is seen in diabetes mellitus and during pregnancy.

Specific gravity

Specific gravity measures the kidney functionality in the means of concentrating urine. It can also be a measure of a patient's hydration status

Normal urine has a specific gravity of 1.005 - 1.025.
Low-level specific gravity can indicate too much fluid intake. It is seen in diabetes insipidus, pyelonephritis, and tubular necrosis.
High specific gravity is due to a low amount of fluid in the blood, which may be due to vomiting or sweat. Also, it occurs in glomerulonephritis, liver or heart failure, nephrotic syndrome.

Protein

Two methods are used to check for protein in the urine—the dipstick and sulfosalicylic acid method.

Albumins are tested and confirmed using dipstick measures, but they cannot trace smaller proteins like microalbumin. However, it is sensitive and highly accurate.

The results are:

- 4+ : 1000 mg/dl or more
- 3+ : 300 mg/dl
- 2+ : 100 mg/dl
- 1+ : 30 mg/dl
- Trace proteinuria: 10 - 30 mg/dl

Sulfosalicylic acid test can test and confirm different types of proteins: Bence-Jones protein, and globulins. Results are:

- 4+ : 1000 mg/dl or more (dense precipitate)
- 3+ : 500 mg/dl (flocculation)
- 2+ : 200 mg/dl (print invisible)
- 1+ : 50 mg/dl (print visible through specimen)
- Traces : 20 mg/dl (slight turbidity)
- 0 : 0 mg/dl (no turbidity)

The average protein level in the urine should not exceed 150 mg/dl. A high protein levels in the urine is an indicator of leukemia, poison, diabetes, heart failure, high blood pressure, or an infection.

Ketones

The three ketones are beta-hydroxybutyric acid, acetone, and acetoacetic acid. They are produced during the metabolism of fat and are excreted through the urine. There should be zero ketones in the urine under normal conditions; however,they are produced and excreted during starvation or diet-related disorders and find their way into the urine. Ketones are mainly found in patients with uncontrolled diabetes.

Nitrites

Normal urine should test negative for nitrites. However, in detecting urine infection, a test for nitrites may be done. This is because some bacteria convert nitrates to nitrites. Some UTI causing bacteria (like streptococcus and staphylococcus) cannot convert nitrates into nitrites. And this is why this test does not always confirm UTI infection. So, the negative result of nitrites in the urine does not rule out UTI.

Bilirubin

Bilirubin is not usually present in large quantities in the blood. So, regular blood should test negative for bilirubin. Notwithstanding, conjugated or water-soluble bilirubin may be excreted in conditions like hepatitis or obstructive hepatobiliary.

Urobilirubin

Certain bacteria convert bilirubin to urobilirubin. This occurs mainly in the intestines and is excreted in the urine. The average level of urobilirubin is 0.5 to 1 mg/dl. Urobilirubin may be increased in liver conditions, or excess hemolysis decreased in obstructive biliary disease and cholestasis.

Human chorionic gonadotropin

Human chorionic gonadotropin is seen during pregnancy and tested about 10 days after pregnancy. It is noticed only in humans and more specifically in women, as the placenta produces it during pregnancy.

Leukocyte esterase test

Leukocyte esterase is released when white blood cells undergo lysis, and the quantity of white blood cells in urines is small, thus, the amount of leukocyte esterase; and regular urine test should be negative for leukocyte esterase. A positive test of leukocyte esterase in the blood is due to an infection, commonly called pyuria. Leukocyte esterase test is used to diagnose some UTIs causing microorganisms that are extremely difficult to grow in standard urine culture, and they include Mycobacteria, among others.

9.2 Microscopic Analysis of Urine

Microscopic analysis is a test to find microscopic elements, like red blood cells, cast, bacteria, yeast cells, crystals, squamous cells, and white blood cells.

Blood

The appearance of blood-urine is hematuria, and it demands a lot of evaluation to know the cause and clinical treatments. Normally, blood should not be present in the urine, and various reasons are due to malignancies, urinary tract infection, kidney stone, and glomerulonephritis.

Red blood cells

The amount of ERT in the blood should not exceed 2 RBCs per HPF. Any amount that is more than this indicates the presence of microscopic hematuria.

White blood cells

White blood cells, on an average level, should be less than 2 to 5 WBCs per HPF. Abnormality in white blood cells shows current and past information about the infection and contamination of the specimen.

Urinary lymphocytes indicate tubulointerstitial renal diseases, and urinary eosinophils indicate acute interstitial nephritis.

Casts

Casts are secreted by the renal tubular cells. Casts are cylindrical particles, which are coagulated proteins, and are seen in different specs in the urine.

Type of Cast	**Differential condition**
Granular cast	Acute tubular necrosis
Fatty acids	Nephrotic syndrome
Hyaline casts	Less than (5) in healthy individuals, and increased during an exercise
Red cell casts	Glomerulonephritis Vasculitis
Waxy casts	Advanced renal failure

Epithelial cells

Usually, the epithelial cells of the urethra and bladder may be seen in the urine, and this should not go past 15 - 20 cells per HPF. Any deviation or increase in cells is due to infections, or other clinical significances, and must be monitored when noticed in a patient.

Crystals

Crystals are the coagulation of dissolved solutes in the urine. It occurs naturally in some states, but it can also be a result of specific infections, which are differentiated by their shapes and composition.

Composition	**Shape**	**Differential condition**
Uric acid	Barrett shape	Tumor lysis syndrome, acute kidney injury Gout
Calcium oxalate	Envelope shaped	Ethylene glycol ingestion, acute kidney injury

Cysteine	Hexagonal	Cystinuria
Magnesium ammonium phosphate and triple phosphate	Coffin lid shaped	Urinary tract infections

9.3 Stool Analysis

The main idea of stool analysis is to diagnose diseases or infections related to gastrointestinal tracts and other system parts. The test is carried out using gross examination, chemical test, microbiological examination, and screening test.

9.3.0 Gross Examination

The stool can be semi-solid and brown, or yellow-green. Any deviations from the standard form may indicate tapeworm, trophozoites, or cysts in the stool.

9.3.1 Synovial fluid examination

Synovial fluid, or joint fluid, has a composition like that of plasma, and it may change due to some inflammation changes in the body.

The fluid is distributed across all joints in the body. Some evaluation is done on the synovial fluid examination, and some are listed below.

Chemical examination

Proteins level: protein level is one-third of the serum; it increases due to hemorrhagic disorder or inflammatory conditions.

Glucose: it may be decreased in conditions like ankylosis, gout, and sepsis. Glucose has the same measure as blood glucose.

Physical examination

Color	**Appearance**
Clear	Normal synovial fluid
Yellow	Osteoarthritis and trauma, mostly non-inflammatory conditions
Dense yellow (with crystal formation and turbidity)	Synovial fluid has a high viscosity, which may decrease in arthritis thus;, due to

	inflammatory conditions
Yellowish green or cloudy	Septic conditions

Microscopic examination

Leukocyte counts are less than 200 cells per ul.
Neutrophils are less than 25% of 200 cells per ul.
The white blood cell counts are raised by non-inflammatory conditions.

9.3.2 Cerebrospinal fluid examination

Cerebrospinal fluid does the work of a shock absorber to the brain, and it gives mechanical cushioning. Moreover, it serves as a transport vehicle to metabolic reactions and maintains homeostasis. The choroid plexus in the ventricles of the brain produces cerebrospinal fluid.

Many CSF analyses are used to test various injuries or infections that are suspected to have elongated to the brain. Some of the approaches are listed below.

Biochemistry

Biochemistry shows the mechanism and biochemical process involved in each component of the brain. And they are summarized below.

Component	Normal range	Differences
Albumin	Serum is 500 times higher than albumin	Damage blood-brain barrier
Glutamine	8 - 18 mg/dl	Reye syndrome Liver disease
Glucose	60 - 80 % in plasma 45 - 80 mg/dl	Meningitis reduces
Lactate	< 20 - 25 mg/dl	Elevated in trauma, meningitis, and intracranial hemorrhage

Microscopic tests

Conditions like lymphocytosis increased neutrophils and monocytes, are studied under the microscope using the microscopic test as follows:

Monocytosis: it shows changes in intracranial hemorrhage, CNS malignancies, and chronic meningitis.

Lymphocytosis: it shows changes in Guillain-Barré syndrome, meningitis, neurocysticercosis, and multiple sclerosis.

Increased neutrophils: includes cerebral infarction, acute meningitis, brain abscess, and previous lumbar puncture.

Gross appearance

A typical cerebrospinal fluid is clear and colourless. Any deviation means the presence of an infection or disease. Some of the common infections, in relation to their appearances, are:

- Infectious meningitis appears as turbid or milky CSF
- Cloudy CSF is linked to increased protein content caused by changes in the blood-brain barrier.
- Brain bleed, melanosarcoma, melanoma tumors, and kernicterus appears as xanthochromic/colored CSF

9.3.3 Chemical Test

Test for reducing sugar

A test for reducing sugar is the lactose test. Lactose is present in newborns who cannot convert lactose to glucose and galactose due to enzyme-lactase deficiency. The test also shows the presence of colic and a failure to thrive, and this indicates the presence of lactose intolerance.

Stool pH test

The typical stool pH is 7 to 7.5. Deviation from this trend means an infection, or presence of other substances. If the pH is below 5.6 means carbohydrate malabsorption.

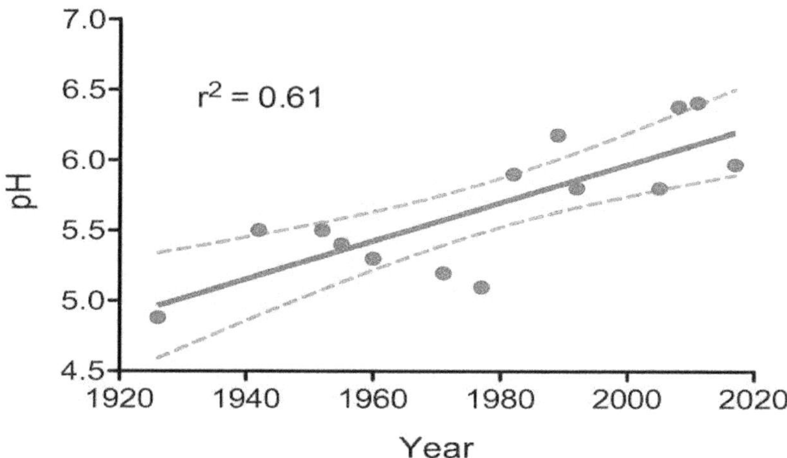

Test for urobilinogen

Urobilinogen is excreted from the body through the urine and stool. Urobilinogen is formed from conjugated bilirubin in the liver. The average excreted value of urobilinogen in the stool is 50 - 300 mg/day. Deviation from these values is noticed in patients with liver disease, oral antibiotic therapy, and biliary tract obstruction.

Test for steatorrhea

Steatorrhea is the measure of dietary fat absorption. When fat is not absorbed in the body, it leads to bile duct obstruction, intestinal disease, and pancreatic insufficiency.

The absorption measures are valued as: decreased serum levels show lower carotene absorption, osteomalacia shows reduced vitamin D absorption, and low vitamin K absorption shows hemorrhage.

The test is carried out over a 72-hour test for stool.

Standard < 5 g per day
Equivocal 5 - 7 g
Steatorrhea > 7 g

Steatorrhea test can also be carried out using a microscope of fat-stained stool.

Fecal osmotic gap:

Fecal osmotic gap calculates the concentration of electrolytes in the stool; in osmotic diarrhea it is more than 150 moan/kg. And in secretory diarrhea, it is less than 50 moan/kg.

http://www.etymonline.com/index.php?term=urinalysis&allowed_in_frame=0

http://labtestsonline.org/understanding/features/ref-ranges/start/6

http://www.mayoclinic.org/diseases-conditions/urine-color/basics/causes/con-20032831

Chapter 10: Arterial Blood Gases Evaluation

Blood vessel-blood gas concentration fundamentally assesses the measure of gases – oxygen and carbon dioxide, in the patient's blood. There are five segments of blood vessel blood gases, which are as per the following:

LOOK AT THE CHART BELOW TO DETERMINE THE EVALUATION OF ABNORMAL VALUES:

Test	Normal	↓ Value	↑ Value
pH	7.35-7.45	Acidosis	Alkalosis
pCO2	35-45	Alkalosis	Acidosis
HCO3	22-26	Acidosis	Alkalosis
p02	80-100	Hypoxemia	02 Therapy
Sa02	95-100%	Hypoxemia	——

The halfway pressing factor of carbon dioxide ($PaCO_2$)

This value demonstrates the measure of carbon dioxide disintegrated in the blood. This is an impression of how well carbon dioxide leaves the blood and moves out of the body through the lung alveoli.

The partial pressing factor of oxygen (PaO_2)

This value shows the critical factor, or measure, of oxygen broke up in the blood vessel blood. This reflects how well the oxygen can move from the lungs' alveoli into the circulation system to arrive at the tissues.

Bicarbonate (HCO_3)

Bicarbonate is a compound that is normally present in the blood. It works as support and keeps up the blood at homeostatic pH.

pH

This value estimates the corrosive base equilibrium of the blood.
Blood is slightly alkaline and has a pH of 7.35 to 7.45. In the event that this value decreases, the patient may have acidosis, while, in the event that it increases, the patient may have alkalosis.

Oxygen immersion (SaO2)

This value fundamentally gauges the convergence of oxygen in hemoglobin. This also evaluates the measure of oxygen in the blood, while PaO2 estimates the centralization of oxygen in plasma. A synopsis of the typical scopes of blood vessel blood gas parts is recorded underneath.

Evaluating acid-base disorder

To accurately analyze infections, sequential ABGs may typically be taken. It is critical to recall that, in an ordinary ABG, pH and PaCO2 move in inverse ways, HCO3 and PaCO2 move similarly. Utilizing blood vessel-blood gases to assess corrosive base problems: ABG is principally used to determine corrosive base issues. Corrosive base problems might be metabolic, respiratory, or blended issues.

The accompanying focuses should be remembered while attempting to decipher corrosive base issues:

- Change in PaCO2 levels is characteristic of a respiratory issue, while a change in HCO3 is demonstrative of a metabolic issue.
- The abbreviation ROME (Respiratory Opposite, Opposite, Metabolic Equal) merits recollecting here.
- A low pH demonstrates acidosis, while a high pH shows alkalosis.

In metabolic problems, the pay is finished by the lungs, which attempt to discharge carbon dioxide in acidosis (low PaCO2), and tries to hold it in alkalosis (high PaCO2). Anion Gap: it's the distinction between the essential estimated cations (Na+, K+) and anions (Cl-, HCO3-) available in the blood.

In the event that the pH and paCO2 move in inverse ways (one worth increment from typical during further reductions, or the other way around), the essential issue is respiratory. In the event that both pH and HCO3 move a similar way (the two qualities are higher, and both are lower than typical), the essential issue is metabolic.

In uncompensated problems, the HCO_3 stays normal for respiratory issues while $PaCO_2$ stays normal for metabolic problems. Notwithstanding, typically, the body attempts to make up for the strange blood pH by trying to tackle it.

In respiratory problems, compensation is brought by the kidneys, which will hold more bicarbonate in acidosis (expanding blood HCO_3), and discharge more bicarbonate in alkalosis (diminished blood HCO_3).

$AG = (Na^+ + K^+) – (Cl^- - HCO_3^-)$ Normal AG is 3 – 11 mEq/l A high anion hole, particularly more than 20 mEq/l, might be characteristic of metabolic acidosis.

ABGs are drawn for an assortment of reasons. These may incorporate worry for:

- Injury
- Uncontrolled diabetes
- Lung Failure
- Kidney Failure
- Asthma

- Ongoing Obstructive Pulmonary Disease (COPD)
- Stun
- Medication Overdose
- Metabolic Disease
- To check if lung condition medicines are working
- Metabolic confusion
- Synthetic Poisoning
- Discharge

In patients with metabolic acidosis, an overabundance of corrosive or loss of base is available. This causes the HCO_3:H_2CO_3 ratio and pH to fall while no change happens in $paCO_2$–uncompensated metabolic acidosis.

Anion gap

For over 40 years, the AG hypothesis has been utilized by clinicians to misuse the idea of electro-neutrality. It has been developed as a significant device for assessing the corrosive base issue. Anion gap is the distinction between the charges of plasma anions and cations, determined from the contrast between the regularly estimated convergence of the serum cations (Na^+ and K^+) and anions ($Cl^-$and HCO_3^-). Since electro-neutrality should be kept up, the distinction mirrors the unmeasured particles. Regularly, this distinction, or the gap, is filled by the less active acids (A^-), and less active phosphates, sulfates, and lactates.

When the AG is more noteworthy than that created by the albumin protein and phosphate, different anions (e.g., lactates and ketones) should be higher than typical fixation.

Anion gap = $(Na^+ + K^+) - [Cl^- + HCO_3^-]$

Due to its low and tight extracellular focus, K^+ is frequently discarded from the computation.

The essential issue with AG is its dependence on the utilization of the ordinary reach created by the albumin protien and less significantly phosphate, the degree of which might be strange in basically sick patients. Since these anions are not solid, their charges will be modified by changes in pH.

Serum protein and phosphate

Typical AG = 2{albumin(gm/L)} + 0.5 {phosphate (mg/dL)}

Corrosive base status

In Acidemic state - Anion gap diminishes by 1-3

In Alkalemic state - Anion gap increments by 2-5

Principal clinical employments of the anion gap.

For flagging, the presence of metabolic acidosis and affirm different discoveries.

Reasons for metabolic acidosis: High AG versus normal AG metabolic acidosis. In an inorganic metabolic acidosis (e.g., because of HCl imbuement), the injected Cl-replaces HCO_3^-, and the AG stays normal. In a natural acidosis, the lost bicarbonate is supplanted by the corrosive anion, which isn't ordinarily estimated. This implies that the AG is expanded.

Giving help with evaluating the biochemical seriousness of the acidosis and follow the reaction to treatment.
In the patients with metabolic alkalosis, there is an abundance of base or a deficiency of acidic, which causes the HCO_3^-:H_2CO_3 proportion and pH to rise, yet with no change happening in $paCO_2$, which is called uncompensated metabolic alkalosis. In any case, the kidney has a considerable ability to discharge abundance bicarbonate; thus, for supporting the metabolic alkalosis, the raised HCO_3^-focus should be kept up through strange renal maintenance of HCO_3^-.

Compensatory respiratory acidosis might be set apart to the point that pCO_2 may ascend higher than 55 mmHg. Expected $paCO_2$ is determined as $paCO_2 = [0.7 \times HCO_3^- + 21] \pm 2$ or $40 + [0.7 \Delta HCO_3]$. This is called remunerated metabolic alkalosis.

The vast majority of the patients with metabolic alkalosis can be treated with chloride particles as NaCl (saline responsive) instead of KCl. When NaCl is given, Cl^-particles are provided; thus, the blood volume increments and the discharge of aldosterone diminishes. Along these lines, extreme urinary loss of K^+ and unnecessary reabsorption of HCO_3 stops. When metabolic alkalosis happens because of the impacts of excessive aldosterone or different mineralocorticoids, the patient doesn't react to NaCl and requires KCl.

Given the urinary chloride, metabolic alkalosis is partitioned into:

- Chloride responsive or extracellular volume exhaustion (urinary chloride < 20)
- Retching
- Diuretic
- Post hypercapnic
- Persistent the runs
- Choride safe (urinary chloride > 20)
- Serious potassium exhaustion
- Mineralocorticoid abundance Primary hyperaldosteronism, Cushing's Syndrome, Ectopic ACTH
- Auxiliary hyperaldosteronism–Renovascular illness, threatening hypertension, CHF, cirrhosis

Approach to blended turmoil

Blended metabolic aggravations (e.g., high AG from diabetic ketoacidosis and normal AG from the runs) can be recognized utilizing the connection between AG and HCO3, known as the gap proportion. The proportion of progress in anion gap (ΔAG) to change in HCO3 (ΔHCO3-). When hydrogen particles aggregate in blood, the abatement in serum HCO3- is comparable to the increment in AG, and the increment in AG abundance/HCO3-shortage proportion is in harmony, i.e., unadulterated expansion in AG metabolic acidosis. At the point when a typical AG acidosis is available, the ratio approaches zero. When a blended acidosis is general (high AG + specific AG), the gap proportion shows the overall commitment of each kind to the acidosis. In the event that it is <1, at that point, it proposes that there is a typical AG metabolic acidosis related to it and if >2, it recommends that there is related metabolic acidosis.

Rules for fast clinical translation of ABG

At the moment we need to make an appropriate step towards the assessment of blood gas and corrosive base aggravations in the body, the following plan is recommended:

Take a gander at pH - < 7.40 - Acidosis; > 7.40 – Alkalosis.

In the event that pH shows acidosis, at that point, take a gander at $paCO_2$and HCO_3^-.

In the event that $paCO_2$is ↑, at that point, it is essential respiratory acidosis.

To decide if it is intense or ongoing.

$\Delta H^+/\Delta paCO_2 < 0.3$–ongoing.

>0.8–intense.

0.3-0.8–intense on ongoing.

Ascertain pay by the individual techniques.

Intense: [HCO_3^-] ↑ by 1 mEq/L for each 10 mmHg ↑ in $paCO_2$ over 40.

In the event that $paCO_2$↓ and $HCO_3^-$is likewise ↓→ essential metabolic acidosis.

Compute expected $paCO_2$ as follows:

$paCO_2 = [1.5 \times HCO_3 + 8] \pm 2$ metabolic acidosis in particular.

paCO2 < anticipated paCO2→ accompanying respiratory alkalosis.

paCO2 > anticipated paCO2→ attendant respiratory acidosis.

If HCO3-is ↓, at that point, AG ought to be analyzed.

In the event that AG is unaltered →, at that point, it is hyperchloremic metabolic acidosis.

If AG is ↑ →, at that point, it is wide AG acidosis.

Check gap proportion

ΔAG/Δ HCO3-= 1, unadulterated expanded AG metabolic acidosis.

<1 typical anion hole metabolic acidosis.

>2 related metabolic acidoses.

In the event that pH demonstrates alkalosis, at that point, take a gander at HCO3-and paCO2.

In the event that paCO2is ↓ →, at that point, it is essential respiratory alkalosis.

Regardless of whether it is intense or ongoing (with a similar equation as above).

Ascertain remuneration by the particular strategies:

Intense: [HCO_3^-]↓ by 2 mEq/L for each 10 mmHg.

↓ In $paCO_2$below 40.

Persistent: [HCO_3^-] ↓ by 5 mEq/L each.

10mmHg ↓ in $paCO_2$ under 40.

In the event that $paCO_2$ ↑ and HCO_3^-additionally ↑ →, at that point, it is essential metabolic alkalosis.

Ascertain the normal paCO2

$paCO_2 = [0.7 \times HCO_3^- + 21] \pm 2$ Or $40 + [0.7\ \Delta HCO_3]$ → metabolic alkalosis as it were

$paCO_2$ < anticipated $paCO_2$ → accompanying respiratory alkalosis.

$paCO_2$ > anticipated $paCO_2$ → accompanying respiratory acidosis.

Check urinary chloride

If urinary chloride < 20 → chloride responsive or ECV consumption.

If urinary chloride > 20→ chloride safe.

If pH is typical, ABG might be an ordinary or blended problem.

↑$paCO_2$ and ↓HCO_3^-→ respiratory and metabolic acidosis.

(b) ↓$paCO_2$ and↑ HCO_3^-→ respiratory and metabolic alkalosis.

Figure % distinction ($\Delta HCO_3^-/HCO_3^-$and $\Delta paCO_2/paCO_2$) to see which is prevailing confusion.

The most effective method to Interpret an ABG

The primary value a medical caretaker should take a gander at is the pH to decide whether the patient is in the normal level, above, or beneath. If a patient's pH > 7.45, the patient is in alkalosis. If < 7.35, the patient is in acidosis. Remember, the lower the pH number, the higher the acidic level in the body. What is more, even with an ordinary pH level, acidosis or alkalosis may, in any case, be available, as the body can remunerate to adjust the pH.

Then, inspect the PaCO2. This will decide whether the blood gas adjustments are because of the respiratory framework or metabolically determined. In blend with the HCO3, the medical caretaker will want to understand the blood gas completely.

The following is an explanation that contains the various qualities and deciding whether the reason is respiratory or metabolic-driven. If, how much, the patient is making up for the pH. This will empower the clinical group to treat the patient sufficiently.

http://www.patient.info/doctor/Arterial-Blood-Gases-Indications-and-Interpretation.htm

http://clinchem.aaccjnls.org/content/47/10/1845.long

https://web.archive.org/web/19980424232639/http://pathcuric1.swmed.edu/PathDemo/NRRT.htm

https://doi.org/10.3109%2F00365519609088622

Chapter 11: Infection Serological Tests

When disease attacks the body, antibodies are created as a safeguard instrument against these organic entities. Serological tests are utilized to evaluate the estimations of these antibodies that are available in the blood. They can be used for a wide assortment of illnesses. The translation of serological test outcomes is genuinely straightforward for a medical caretaker. If the test shows that no antibodies are available, there is no contamination. In the event that there are antibodies present, it could demonstrate an ebb and flow contamination, a past one, or once in a while, presence of immune system infection. The outcomes should consistently be connected with clinical discoveries. While talking about all the serological tests is past the extent of this book, the main ones needed for medical attendants are illustrated in this part.

Serological markers for hepatitis B

There are a few serological markers for hepatitis B contamination; these incorporate HBsAg, enemies of HBs, HBeAg, against HBe, and hostile to HBc. HBsAg is the main serological marker for hepatitis B contamination.

It shows up in the serum 1 to 10 weeks after openness and endures for over a half year. Enemies of Hbs are distinguished in patients who have gone through inoculation.

Test for typhoid

Widal test: This test examins two distinct sorts of antibodies – H-agglutinin and O-agglutinin. H-agglutinin tests past disease, while O-agglutinin tests dynamic contamination. A titer of more than 1:160 is viewed as sure. Different tests:

- Bacterial diseases, for example, Brucellosis Syphilis Viruses, which could include, Measles-Rubella Cytomegalovirus and herpes infection
- Fungal contaminations, for example, aspergillosis Parasite contaminations, which could include amoebiasis.

Tests for HIV

The human immunodeficiency virus causes an illness called AIDS. Antibodies to HIV will grow in 90-95% people in a quarter of a year of openness, and 99% people inside a half year of transparency. There are two serological tests for HIV. The ELISA test is utilized for screening purposes, while the Western smudge test is corroborative. A reference estimation of under 1.0 is viewed as unfavorable.

CD4 check: The HIV infection will, in general, obliterate the CD4 T-cells, so it is essential to audit the tally of these cells intermittently. The typical scope of CD4 cells in a solid body: 500 cells for each cubic mm of blood. A measure lower than 200/mm3 is analyzed as AIDS. CD4 rate, which decides the proportion of these cells to add up to white platelets, gives a more precise picture. Viral burden test measures the number of infectious particles per milliliter of blood. A viral burden under 50 is supposed to be imperceptible. When a patient is beginning to exhibit hostility to retroviral treatment, this value is utilized to screen the patient's reaction to medicine.

Any patient who tests positive for HIV will require more lab testing, because of the very incapacitating nature of the infection. The accompanying tests should be acted on in these patients.

11.1 Bacteremia and septic shock workup

In the anti-microbial period, most contaminations are not hazardous. In any case, in uncommon instances, malign life forms can enter the circulation system and can undermine any form of protection. The accompanying tests are done when bacteremia or septic stun is suspected: Complete blood check: including hemoglobin, white platelet tally, and differential tally.

WBC of more than 15 for every histopathological field is demonstrative of bacteremia. Platelet tally, alongside PT and APTT, is vital to screen spread intravascular coagulation. Serum electrolytes to survey for parchedness and acidosis. Glucose to screen for hyperglycemia. Renal capacities and liver capacity tests.

11.2 Utilization of Infection Serological test

Bonding medication

O positive blood classification: the patient's red cells are agglutinated by Anti-D (hostile to Rh factor) antisera, yet not against An and hostile to B antisera. The patient's plasma agglutinates type An and B red cells.

Blood composing is commonly performed utilizing serologic strategies. The antigens on an individual's red platelets, which decide their blood classification, are distinguished using reagents that contain antibodies, called **antisera**. When the antibodies tie to red platelets that express the comparing antigen, they influence red platelets to bunch together (**agglutinate**), which can be distinguished outwardly.

The individual's blood bunch antibodies can be characterized by adding plasma to cells that express the relating antigen and noticing the agglutination reactions.

Other serologic strategies utilized in bonding medication incorporate *cross-matching* and the immediate and backhanded anti-globulin tests.

The backhanded anti-globulin test is utilized to screen for antibodies that could cause bonding responses and distinguish specific blood bunch antigens.
In microbiology, serologic tests are used to decide whether an individual has antibodies against a particular microorganism or to identify antigens related to a microorganism in an individual's sample. Serologic tests are precious for creatures that are hard to culture by routine research facility techniques, similar to Treponema pallidum (the causative specialist of syphilis) or viruses.

Cross-matching is performed before a blood bonding to guarantee that the patient blood is viable. It includes adding the patient's plasma to the contributor platelets and noticing for agglutination reactions. The direct anti-globulin test is performed to recognize if antibodies are bound to red platelets inside the individual's body, which is unusual and can happen in conditions like hemolytic sickness of the infant, bonding reactions, and immune system hemolytic iron deficiency.

Antibodies against a microorganism in a patients' blood show that they have been presented to that microbe. Most serologic tests measure one of two sorts of antibodies: immunoglobulin M (IgM) and immunoglobulin G (IgG). IgM is delivered in high amounts not long after an individual is presented to the microorganism, and creation decays rapidly from that point. IgG is likewise created on principle openness, however not as fast as IgM. On resulting openings, the antibodies produced are basically IgG, and they stay available for use for a drawn-out period of time.

This influences the understanding of serology results: a positive outcome for IgG and a negative outcome for IgM proposes that the individual may have been tainted or vaccinated before. In contrast, a positive effect for IgM recommends that an individual is right now, or as of late, contaminated. The measure of immunizer in every example (neutralizer titer) is analyzed, and an altogether higher measure of IgG in the recuperating example recommends an actual disease rather than past exposure. False, contrary outcomes for counteracting agent testing can happen in immunosuppressed individuals. They produce lower measures of antibodies and in individuals who get antimicrobial medications from the get-go over the span of the infection.

Counteracting agent testing for irresistible infections is regularly done in two stages: after recuperation (gaining strength stage) and during the underlying sickness (intense stage).

https://archive.org/details/sherrismedicalmi00ryan

Sherris Medical Microbiology (4th ed.). McGraw Hill. pp. 247–9. ISBN 978-0-8385-8529-0.

Linne & Ringsrud's Clinical Laboratory Science - E-Book: The Basics and Routine Techniques. Elsevier Health Sciences. pp. 586–95, 543, 556. ISBN 978-0-323-37061-5.

Chapter 12: Other Tests

Alpha – 1 antitrypsin

This protein restrains tissue harm that is brought about by trypsin, elastin, and different proteases. *Ordinary qualities:* 20 – 50 μmol/l Alpha-1 antitrypsin lack might be inherent. It is related to the advancement of beginning stage emphysema and neonatal hepatitis, which may advance cirrhosis.

Any provocative cycle in the body can cause expanded levels of this catalyst. Angiotensin changing over chemical: This catalyst assumes a part in vasoconstriction by aiding rennin from the kidneys convert into angiotensin. It like this brings about vasoconstriction and expanded pulse.

Typical worth: 23 – 57 U/l The levels of this catalyst might be expanded in sarcoidosis, Gaucher's illness, hyperthyroidism, psoriasis, amyloidosis, and histoplasmosis. Expanded levels of this compound are utilized for diagnosing sarcoidosis in blend with different modalities like radiology and histopathology C-receptive protein: This is an intense stage serum protein that assumes a significant part in contamination and aggravation. *Typical worth:* < 5mg/ml; however, it expands 100-1000 overlap during aggravation or injury.

This test is done when the incendiary cycle is suspected in the body, e.g., immune system infections, fundamental lupus erythematosus. This test can be joined with ESR to preclude provocative reasons for ESR increment. Sequential trials of this protein are likewise done to screen progressing fiery interaction.

Erythrocyte sedimentation rate (ESR): Erythrocyte sedimentation rate shows how much aggravation is available in the body. This test gauges the speed at which RBC tumble to the lower part of a test tube. This test is demonstrated in Muscle compressions Unexplained fevers Unexplained unclear side effects Certain kinds of joint pain Normal reach fluctuates relying upon the strategy, age, and sex.

As indicated by the Westergren strategy: Adults Men under 50: lower than 15 mm/hr. Men over 50: lower than 20 mm/hr. Ladies under 50: lower than 20 mm/hr. Ladies over 50: lower than 30 mm/hr. Youngsters Newborn: 0 – 2 mm/hr. Infant to pubescence: 3 – 13 mm/hr. This test can be utilized to follow bone contaminations, provocative sicknesses, immune system problems, a few sorts of joint inflammation, and tissue demise. Though the outcome is characteristic, it isn't decisive with respect to the conclusion. One needs to affirm the determination through different tests. Ailments connected to irregular outcomes include kidney infection, sickliness, pregnancy, tumors, thyroid illness, and so forth.

Individuals with immune system issues have a higher rate of expanded ESR. Normal models incorporate lupus and rheumatoid joint inflammation. Different models are essential macroglobulinemia, hypersensitive vasculitis, hyperfibrinogenemia, polymyalgia rheumatica, monster cell arteritis, and necrotizing vasculitis. Irregularities in the ESR rates could emerge from different conditions. Expanded rates may happen because of bone diseases, rheumatic fever, tuberculosis, foundational contamination, heart (or heart valve) diseases, and serious skin diseases. Lower rates can happen within sight of hyperviscosity, congestive cardiovascular breakdown, sickle cell paleness, or leukemia.

Rheumatoid factor

This is an autoantibody delivered in rheumatoid joint pain. Typical worth: < 25 IU/l The blood level of this is expanded in rheumatoid joint inflammation, and hence this test is utilized for the finding of this immune system illness. High levels of this factor show a more forceful infection. The blood levels can be observed in patients with known rheumatoid joint inflammation to manage treatment conventions. Markers for strong dystrophy: Patients with solid dystrophy regularly show anomalous rises in the accompanying markers: a) Lactic dehydrogenase b) Aldolase c) Phosphohexose isomerase d) Glutamic-oxalacetic transaminase

This sort of rising of the compound movement is basic in those with intense cerebral vascular mishaps, yet not found in other neurological issues.

https://portlandpress.com/bioscirep/article-abstract/9/2/129/56650/Alpha1-antitrypsin-Structure-function-and?redirectedFrom=fulltext

https://www.sciencedirect.com/science/article/abs/pii/S0167483899002642?via%3Dihub

Conclusion

As much as we have discussed, that there are many laboratory tests into the practice of successful medical procedures, it is important that all the tests are mere significant approaches to other practices, and this is the basic of other treatments. Examination of the tests and results of laboratory procedures serve as the backbone to other investigations. And if the values are back to normal, it is important to carry out a test or further monitoring on the patient to ascertain that the condition is perfectly ok as the condition demands.

Many approaches may be suitable for a single test. Notwithstanding, the necessary test should be done with an absolute mind that cares for all the processes involved.

It is mandatory to memories all the values ranges listed above. Nevertheless, it is beneficial to know or to have the standards values references to check in the crucial times.

Wish you a wonderful journey in your medical world!

www.ingramcontent.com/pod-product-compliance
Ingram Content Group UK Ltd.
Pitfield, Milton Keynes, MK11 3LW, UK
UKHW021909190726
13853UKWH00002B/580